Leadership and Management for Doctors in Training

D0077288

Leadership and Management for Doctors in Training

A PRACTICAL GUIDE

STEPHEN GILLAM

General Practitioner, Luton
Director of Public Health Teaching
School of Clinical Medicine, University of Cambridge

With contributions from
PAUL COSFORD

Interim Executive Director of Health Protection Services
Health Protection Agency

Foreword by
SIR BRUCE KEOGH

NHS Medical Director

Radcliffe Publishing
London • New York

Radcliffe Publishing Ltd
33–41 Dallington Street
London
EC1V 0BB
United Kingdom

www.radcliffepublishing.com
Electronic catalogue and worldwide online ordering facility.

British Library Cataloguing in Publication Data

A catalogue record for this book is available from the British Library.

ISBN-13: 978 184619 416 0

Typeset by Pindar NZ, Auckland, New Zealand
Printed and bound by Cadmus Communications, USA

Contents

Foreword

The quality of leadership and management define the difference between excellence and mediocrity – success and failure – for all organisations. In my view, good leaders inspire others and are able to align them towards a common goal through a clear vision. Good managers, on the other hand, simplify and streamline the way organisations work to achieve their goals and maximise potential. These two are quite different functions. Not all leaders are good managers but most effective managers are also good leaders.

In healthcare provider organisations, the quality of clinical leadership always underpins the difference between exceptional and adequate clinical services which, in aggregate, determine their overall effectiveness, safety and reputation. Similarly, effective clinical leadership in commissioning organisations drives up clinical quality for the whole health economy. So, good clinical leadership is not an end in itself but a means to achieving high performing healthcare systems.

Over 1.4 million people work in our NHS which is undergoing enormous change with the aim of giving more managerial and leadership responsibility to clinicians. Young doctors are inspired by good clinicians: those who are intellectually adept, who bring forensic scrutiny to their diagnostic and therapeutic routines, who are kind to their patients and exhibit a comprehensive mixture of compassion and professionalism. Such doctors may have no overt managerial inclinations, yet they are highly influential and essential leaders if the NHS is to flourish.

Doctors also seek leadership from medical royal colleges and the specialist associations with whom they identify on matters of clinical quality, standards of care and training of the next generation.

In other words, clinical leadership across the NHS may take many forms ranging from frontline leaders who provide excellent service through a spectrum of clinical innovators and academics, to those who provide leadership through their professional bodies or through managerial involvement at various levels in their employing institution.

Successful medical managers are usually, but not always, experienced clinicians with good 'people skills', who look outside the boundaries of their own specialty, who exhibit passion through positivity and perseverance and are prepared to take reasonable risks to achieve their goals. Perhaps most importantly they know how to engage colleagues and effect change. They understand the core principles of management.

This admirable book is aimed at young clinicians and invites them, through a series of vignettes and issues coupled with practical theory, to enter the world of management. I hope that everyone who reads this book will accept that invitation, because it is only through effective service design, management and change that we can practise medicine in the way and in the environment that is best for both patients and clinicians.

Professor Sir Bruce Keogh
NHS Medical Director
February 2011

About the author

Stephen Gillam is a GP at the Lea Vale Medical Group in Luton and Director of Undergraduate Public Health Teaching at the University of Cambridge School of Clinical Medicine. Previously, he was Director of Primary Care at The King's Fund, where he was heavily involved in charting the impact of health policy under New Labour and developing medical managers. He is an honorary consultant at the Cambridgeshire Primary Care Trust and a visiting professor at the University of Bedfordshire.

CONTRIBUTOR

Paul Cosford is Interim Executive Director of Health Protection Services at the Health Protection Agency, and previously was Regional Director of Public Health in the East of England. He has extensive experience of medical management, including addressing professional performance and patient safety concerns in acute, mental health and primary care. He is an Honorary Senior Fellow at the University of Cambridge and has a particular interest in quality and safety of healthcare.

Paul Cosford is co-author of Chapters 8 and 12, and also offered comments and suggestions to the author on the rest of the book.

To many manager colleagues – past, present or future – who have shaped our understanding and practice of healthcare.

Acknowledgements: Jenny Amery, Jennifer Dixon, Philippa Drew, John Lawler, Richard Lewis, Bernie Naughton, Paul Tracey, Julian Tudor Hart, Diane Plamping, Anne Yardumian.

Introduction

While your focus is on learning how to manage patients, all doctors work in organisations. In general practices and hospitals, responsibilities for leading and managing within the organisation are shared with other colleagues but, as doctors, you have broader legal duties than other health professionals. You have an intrinsically different role within healthcare and, of course, you share responsibility for the quality of services provided. This book aims to make you a more effective leader and manager.

BOX A Scenarios

Mary P was 71 years old with end-stage chronic renal failure due to diabetes. Other co-morbidities precluded her from renal transplant surgery. Over months during which her appeals for surgery were turned down, the junior doctor watched her inexorable decline. Mary eventually refused peritoneal dialysis and died in uraemic coma.

Shortly after being injected with contrast medium by a junior doctor as part of a radiological investigation, Roy P suffered an anaphylactic reaction, myocardial infarction and death. At post mortem, this 67-year-old man was found to have unknown ischaemic heart disease. The junior doctor concerned was comforted by colleagues after this distressing event but no further action was taken.

A senior registrar in obstetrics and gynaecology, Peter L, was known to be a heavy drinker. When 'on call', he was frequently to be found in the hospital bar consuming alcohol with colleagues. A junior doctor wondered whether he was fit to operate on these occasions.

These commonplace encounters were experienced by the author within three months of qualifying. How, he wondered, had the decision to refuse his patient a renal transplant – thereby terminating her life – been taken? The profession had unconsciously closed ranks but should more have been done after Roy's death to learn from these events and inform his family? Was it appropriate that an otherwise competent colleague should be drinking on duty?

Health professionals and junior doctors may feel powerless to influence systems and working routines in their place of work. However, we share responsibility for the quality of services our team delivers. Knowing what systems exist and how most constructively to influence them is an essential part of medical practice.

This is affirmed by the General Medical Council in their blueprint for training, which states that graduates should 'demonstrate awareness of the role of doctors as managers'.[1] The relevant learning outcomes are listed in Box B. While management training for senior medical leaders within the National Health Service (NHS) has long been available, an introduction to these areas for students has only recently been accorded a priority for students. How, when and, indeed, whether student doctors need management training remains a matter of earnest debate but this book addresses these learning needs.

BOX B Doctors' duties as professionals in protecting patients and improving care[1]

'Graduates will
(a) Place patients' needs and safety at the centre of the care process.
(b) Deal effectively with uncertainty and change.
(c) Understand the framework in which medicine is practised in the UK, including: the organisation, management and regulation of healthcare provision; the structures, functions and priorities of the NHS; and the roles of, and relationships between, the agencies and services involved in protecting and promoting individual and population health.
(d) Promote, monitor and maintain health and safety in the clinical setting, understanding how errors can happen in practice, applying the principles of quality assurance, clinical governance and risk management to medical practice, and understanding responsibilities within the current systems for raising concerns about safety and quality.
(e) Understand and have experience of the principles and methods of improvement, including audit, adverse incident reporting and quality improvement, and how to use the results of audit to improve practice.
(f) Respond constructively to the outcomes of appraisals, performance reviews and assessments.
(g) Demonstrate awareness of the role of doctors as managers, including seeking ways to continually improve the use and prioritisation of resources.
(h) Understand the importance of, and the need to keep to, measures to prevent the spread of infection, and apply the principles of infection prevention and control.
(i) Recognise own personal health needs, consult and follow the advice of a suitably qualified professional, and protect patients from any risk posed by own health.
(j) Recognise the duty to take action if a colleague's health, performance or conduct is putting patients at risk.'

Our approach rests on three contentions. First, you have more knowledge and experience in this field than you realise. Most students at one time or another have been involved in leadership and management. Second, 'management' is in many ways a core medical skill rather than a wholly separate field of endeavour. Students of healthcare have many opportunities for observation and reflection on the activities of others, for self-directed study reading around the subject, and for modelling new skills in practice. This book seeks to help you make the most of the opportunities. Our third conviction is that you will thereby continue to develop understanding and skills in these areas over a professional lifetime. The wisest leaders and managers, like the wisest doctors, are continually aware of their limitations and educational needs. The sooner you are aware of your developmental needs, the better you will address them.

> **Q:** Can you think of leadership and management roles you have already undertaken? Performing sports, plays or concerts; doing voluntary work, the Duke of Edinburgh's Award or other formalised schemes, and so forth. List them.

A HISTORICAL DIGRESSION

If one event above all others has transformed medical attitudes and practice in the recent past it is surely the inquiry into charges surrounding paediatric cardiac surgery in Bristol between 1988 and 1995. The case attracted huge public interest. Held in public, it was monitored closely by those parents on whose children the surgeons operated and of whom over 30 had died. Two surgeons were found to have continued to operate despite growing concerns over mortality figures. They did not adequately establish the causes of those results. One of them misled parents about the likely outcomes. The medical chief executive failed to take sufficient action when colleagues voiced anxieties. Many issues were raised by the Bristol inquiry[2] (*see* Box C) and it is fair to say that many positive developments have resulted from these awful events. In how it is monitored and regulated, medical practice has forever 'changed utterly'.[3]

BOX C Concerns identified by the Bristol inquiry

- The absence of clearly understood clinical standards.
- Confusion as to how clinical competence and technical expertise are assessed.
- Unreliable and invalid data used to monitor doctors' personal performance.
- Poor appreciation of the non-clinical factors affecting clinical performance.
- Responsibility of doctors to take prompt, appropriate actions in response to concerns about their own or their colleagues' performance.
- Factors discouraging openness about doctors' personal performance.
- How doctors explain risks to patients.
- Ways people concerned about patients' safety can make their concerns known.

CLINICAL LEADERSHIP

Leadership and management are not, of course, the same thing, though they are often conflated. Doctors' roles as leaders and managers are not ours by right – though they are often assumed. Remember that bright graduates from a host of backgrounds dedicate years to training for health service management. Learn from them. By contrast, doctors are sometimes poor managers; the term 'clinical leadership' can seem oxymoronic!

Leadership skills help doctors become more actively involved in planning and delivery of health services but also support roles in research, education and health politics. Doctors differ significantly from other managers in (usually) continuing to deliver hands-on clinical services. This provides an understanding of how management decisions impact on clinical practice and the care of patients, and can help translate national initiatives into local practice as effectively as possible.

Management competencies are important to us as health professionals for three overriding reasons. They help us to:

➤ improve the efficiency of what we do in helping make best use of always limited resources
➤ ensure systems are in place to monitor and maintain quality of care, the stuff of 'clinical governance', which is concerned with patient safety and quality
➤ cope constructively with change as health services continually evolve and develop.

Many doctors also have satisfying careers in health services management. They wish to influence the wider healthcare system in which their patients are treated. They know how to challenge the status quo to improve care. While the immediacy of individual patient care may be lost, doctor managers often feel that they benefit more patients than they would in full-time clinical practice. After all, if you are frustrated that 'the system' does not enable you to provide the best possible patient care, why not move into a role where you can have greater influence over that system? The opportunities are many, from working on clinical committees within places of work (for example, prescribing formulary committees), joining advisory committees for national organisations producing clinical guidance (such as the National Institute for Health and Clinical Excellence (NICE) appraisal committees), to more formalised management roles such as a being a clinical or medical director in a hospital, or even a chief executive. Indeed, recent years have seen a drive within the NHS to encourage doctors to take up management careers, due to their understanding of how management decisions impact on the care of patients.

THE STRUCTURE OF THIS BOOK

The different elements of this book form a coherent sequence but can be dipped into according to your needs. In other words, the chapters can stand alone. Section I considers the nature of management and leadership. We look at some of the theories and frameworks underlying these concepts. This leads us on to consider important issues such as the culture and structure of organisations and how managers both reflect and shape them.

In Section II, we consider what management and leadership in the NHS look like in practice. We consider how management has evolved in the NHS and some of the enduring challenges for its leaders. Finally, in Section III, we consider your future roles as leaders/managers and how to develop key competencies.

The tone of the book is a practical one. We take you through various scenarios, all of which derive from real-life experience of the author. Along the way we ask you to reflect on your own experience in signposted exercises.

Much management is indeed 'common sense' but the theoretical and research literature relating to the concepts described in these pages is vast. In a short textbook, it is not possible to do justice to all related disciplines. We have tried to distil key frameworks and concepts. Perceptive readers will note inevitable gaps. For the detail of, for example, financial or information management, readers must look to specialist works. The references provide a starting point. For those readers interested in exploring the theoretical literature, Appendix 1 provides further material. Appendix 2 provides more practical resources.

Improving your confidence and ability to address the kind of challenges described in this book is satisfying of itself. Apart from making you more effective as a health professional, individually and when working with others, these skills will enhance your job satisfaction and enrich your career.

REFERENCES

1 General Medical Council. *Tomorrow's Doctors: outcomes and standards for undergraduate medical education.* GMC: London; 2009.

2 Secretary of State for Health. *Learning from Bristol: the report of the public inquiry into children's heart surgery at the Bristol Royal Infirmary, 1984–1995.* Command paper, CM 5207; 2001.

3 Smith R. All changed, changed utterly. *BMJ.* 1998; **316**: 1917–18.

SECTION I

Management and leadership in theory

CHAPTER 1

What is management?

Q: What do you think managers do?

Management in healthcare – like medicine – is about getting things done to improve the care of patients. The majority of doctors work closely alongside managers, but often doctors do not fully understand what managers actually do, and do not see them as partners in improving patient care. This lack of understanding is one source of the tensions that can arise between doctors and managers, but almost all doctors act as managers in some capacity. Consider the practical functions of management listed in the following paragraph. Put simply, doctors wish to deliver high-quality patient care, and this requires doctors to work effectively alongside managers.

Health professionals tend to be 'action-centred', so let's start by considering 10 different practical functions of management when considering an objective that has to be achieved[1] – whether in medicine or in Marks & Spencer.

1 *Defining the task* – it is not enough to have a purpose or aim. A central job of the manager is to break down general aims into specific, manageable tasks.

2 *Planning* – the first step in planning is to be creative: think laterally and use the ideas of others. There are always more options than you originally realised. The second step is to evaluate the options and formulate a working plan. The successful manager is one who can turn a negative situation into a positive one by creative planning.

3 *Briefing* – the plan once made has to be communicated. The ability to run meetings, to make presentations and to write clear instructions is a vital part of a manager's equipment. The five skills of briefing are preparing, clarifying, simplifying, vivifying (making the subject come alive) and being yourself.

4 *Controlling* – the manager should work out what key facts need to be monitored to see if the plan is working, and set standards to measure them against. To control others, you need also to be able to control yourself – for example, managing your time to best effect. (*See* Appendix 2.)

5 *Evaluating* – assessing the consequences of your efforts is a necessary complement

to controlling them. Some form of progress report and/or debriefing meeting is essential. You can't expect people to work hard if they can't see what they are achieving. The people as well as the task need evaluating, and the techniques of appraisal are important tasks for the leader of the team. (*See* Appendix 2.)

6 *Motivating* – simple ways often work best. Recognition, for instance, of someone's efforts, be it by promotion, extra money or, more frequently, by personal commendation, seldom fails. Success motivates people and communicates a new sense of energy and urgency to the group.

7 *Organising* – one of the tasks of a manager is to see that the infrastructure for the work is in place and operating effectively. Nothing annoys staff more than an organisation where nothing works, essential materials are missing and the arrangements and procedures are always being altered. They blame 'the management', although of course the system at fault may also include a lack of clinical leadership to ensure the clinical issues are being addressed appropriately.

8 *Setting an example* – research on successful organisations suggests that key factors are the behaviour, the values, and the standards of their leaders. People take more notice of who you are and what you do than what you say.

9 *Communicating* – clear and effective communication is fundamental to effective management. Clarity and thinking through your objectives and the means for achieving them need to be matched by clarity of the written or spoken word and how these are relayed to those involved in realising your aims.

10 *Housekeeping* – self-care is essential to good management. This includes the challenges of managing your time, coping with pressure – recognising and managing stress – and doing the same for others. (*See* Appendix 2.)

It is useful to think of management as having several different dimensions.

➤ *Principles* – management is about people, securing commitment to shared values, developing staff and achieving results. These help determine the culture of organisations.

➤ *Theories* – management is underpinned by a plethora of different theories and frameworks. These, in turn, shape the language – and jargon – of management.

➤ *Structures* – the way organisations are set up, for example, as bureaucracies, open systems, matrices, networks, and so forth.

➤ *Behaviours* – personal and organisational.

➤ *Techniques* – including communication skills, management by objectives, finance, accounting, planning, marketing, project management and quality assurance.

Understanding management requires knowledge of sociology, political and behavioural sciences, among many other disciplines. Actually applying management skills requires rather less, but some familiarity with the underpinning theory is desirable. Classical management theories evolved out of military theory and were developed as advanced societies industrialised. While they recognised the need to harmonise human aspects of the organisation, problems were essentially seen as technical. Early theories made individuals fit the requirements of the organisation. Later theories borrowing from behavioural psychology and sociology suggest ways in which the organisation needs to fit the requirements of individuals. New management theories tend to layer new (and sometimes contradictory) concepts and ideas on top of older counterparts rather than replace them. The main schools of management theory are summarised in Appendix 1.

KEY CONCEPTS

The so-called 'new public management' is often contrasted with traditional bureau-cracies built on clear structures, accountabilities and chains of command,[2] for healthcare over the last two decades has been significantly shaped by three forces: managerialism, marketisation and governance. In various ways, they can be seen as complementary, with the same ultimate aim of improving efficiency through greater control over healthcare, while making providers (including healthcare professionals) more accountable for their work.[3]

Managerialism

This has involved importing management techniques from the private to the public sector and using these techniques to streamline the delivery of services, minimising unwarranted variation. Some are concerned that healthcare has become proce-duralised and regulated, limiting opportunities for discretionary professional decision-making, epitomised by the growth of guidelines and the rise of evidence-based (cost-conscious) healthcare. However, all healthcare exists in the context of financial limits, requiring the right balance between guidelines based on evidence of best practice and appropriate professional application of those guidelines to individual clinical circumstances. Appropriate management aims to strike that right balance.

Marketisation

This refers to the political process whereby whole areas of social life have been exposed by government to market forces. Services previously designed, delivered and managed by the state have been opened up to competition. In practice, quasi-markets have arisen, in which elements of services are opened to competition from a range of different providers, which may or may not include commercial organisations. Entry and exit from the market may be restricted (hospitals are not allowed to simply fail and close). Services are commissioned (bought) on behalf of groups of users rather than have users pay for their service individually (though personalised health and social care budgets are being piloted). Marketisation required the structural separation of purchasers from providers and much consequential organisational disruption.

Governance

If managerialism and marketisation have helped expose to scrutiny various ineffi-ciencies within health services, they have also highlighted the need for strengthened governance within the National Health Service (NHS). One form of governance is clinical governance, which provides 'the framework through which NHS organisations are accountable for continually improving the quality of their services and safeguarding high standards of care by creating an environment in which excellence in clinical care will flourish'.[4] Modelled on the notion of corporate governance in the private sector, clinical governance is primarily concerned with providing high-quality, safe services and places responsibility for its maintenance on all employees involved in service delivery.[5] Responsibility for clinical quality is central to the manager's role.

CONTEMPORARY CRITIQUES

The underlying ethos is that the market is the most efficient and effective way of delivering services but this is not self-evident from a cursory look at the national experience or international evidence. Managerialism, marketisation and governance have been implemented through top-down command and control. Because markets in health- or social care operate artificially in comparison with open markets, the voices of service users have been not been central in this process. Different amounts of information are often available to the various parties to a transaction and may place them on an unequal footing when striking a deal (or making a decision over healthcare). This 'information asymmetry' is one of the strongest arguments against markets in healthcare.[6]

The systematisation of work routines (specifying the steps to be followed at each stage of the process, e.g. through care pathways and protocols) may be highly appropriate for dealing with regular processes the outcomes of which are certain. However, much healthcare work and outcomes are uncertain and depend to a large extent on the commitment of both the health professional and the service user with their individual perspective, experiences and motivations. Healthcare is not a predictable commodity but is 'co-produced' – that is, it results from interaction between the doctor responding to the patient's account of their problem and the patient's response to the doctor's diagnosis and prescribed treatment.[7]

In summary, the increasing bureaucratisation and top-down control of healthcare work is based on an understanding of organisations and management that involves increasing rationalisation. The judicious use of evidence-based guidelines and standard operating procedures, for example, is highly beneficial. However, too heavy-handed an emphasis on linear approaches may promote a lack of trust in individual workers. As we will see, other models of management and leadership in healthcare are possible and desirable.

KEY POINTS

- Management, like clinical medicine, employs practical skills to improve the care of patients.
- In recent years, management within the NHS has been heavily influenced by ideas and techniques imported from the private sector.

- Healthcare is a complex product and, while market forces can have a beneficial effect on healthcare provision, they cannot be universally applied to improve patient care in all its complexity.

REFERENCES

1 Henderson E, Baker A, Brearley P, *et al. Managing Health Services*. Milton Keynes: Open University; 1991.

2 Hunter DJ. Management and public health. In: Detels R, McEwen J, Beaglehole R, Tanaka H, editors. *Oxford Textbook of Public Health*. 4th ed. Oxford: Oxford University Press; 2002. pp. 921–36.

3 Lawler J, Bilson A. *Social Work Management and Leadership: managing complexity with creativity*. London: Routledge; 2010.

4 Scally G, Donaldson L. Clinical governance and the drive for quality improvement in the new NHS in England. *BMJ*. 1998; **318**: 61–5.

5 Huntington J, Gillam S, Rosen R. Organisational development for clinical governance. *BMJ*. 2000; **321**: 679–82.

6 Arrow K. Uncertainty and the welfare economics of medical care. *Am Econ Rev*. 1963; **53**: 941–73.

7 Harrison S. Co-optation, commodification and the medical model: governing UK medicine since 1991. *Public Administration*. 2009; **87**(2): 184–97.

CHAPTER 2

The nature of leadership

Q: What qualities characterise the leaders you have encountered?

There are a variety of theories on leadership. Much writing and research has produced an exhaustive list of so-called 'trait' or 'dispositional' theories. Early writers tended to suggest that leaders were born, not made, but no one has been able to agree on a particular set of characteristics required. The following are commonly listed as leadership qualities:

➤ above-average intelligence
➤ initiative or the capacity to perceive the need for action and do something about it
➤ self-assurance, courage and integrity
➤ being able to rise above a particular situation and see it in its broader context (the 'helicopter trait')
➤ high energy levels
➤ high achievement career-wise
➤ being goal-directed and being able to think longer term
➤ good communication skills and the ability to work with a wide variety of people.

In other words, almost anything helps and nowadays the notion of core leadership qualities is taken less seriously by management theorists. What is also clear is that the very attributes that might define a leader in one context may be inappropriate in other circumstances. Winston Churchill was famously rejected as prime minister by peacetime Britons.

Modern theories have proposed two types of leadership: transactional and transformational. Transactional leadership attempts to preserve the status quo, while transformational leadership seeks to inspire and engage the emotions of individuals in organisations. They are distinguished by different values, goals and the nature of leader–follower relations. Transactional leadership concentrates on exchanges between leaders and staff, offering rewards for meeting particular standards in performance. Transformational leadership highlights the importance of leaders demonstrating inspirational motivation and concentrates on relationships.[1]

Another popular concept to emerge in more recent literature on leadership is that of 'emotional intelligence'.[2] This is the capacity for recognising our own feelings and those of others, motivating ourselves and managing emotions well in ourselves. In their description of health leadership, Pointer and Sanchez highlight that:[3]

➤ leadership is a process, an action word, which manifests itself in doing
➤ the locus of leadership is vested in an individual
➤ the focus of leadership is those who follow
➤ leaders influence followers – their thoughts, feelings and actions
➤ leadership is done for a purpose: to achieve goals
➤ leadership is intentional, not accidental.

In healthcare increasing consideration is being given to the organisational context within which people work and what is required of a leader in that work situation. For example, following a study of US healthcare workers, Klein and colleagues described four key features of leadership:[4]

1 providing strategic direction
2 instructing team members
3 monitoring team performance
4 providing 'hands-on' assistance when required.

Note that leadership and management are not synonymous. A manager is an individual who holds an office to which roles are attached whereas leadership is one of the roles attached to the office of manager. Just the fact you are in a senior position will not make you a leader, and certainly not an influential one.

POWER

Leaders and managers wield power: the ability to influence others. There are at least four types of power in organisations (*see* Figure 2.1).[5] Two sources are linked directly to the appointment you hold. 'Position power' is that vested in you as an individual by virtue of your role in your organisation. Your job title enables you to give instructions to people in lesser positions and to authorise certain actions. Position power remains highly relevant to a hierarchal organisation such as the National Health Service (NHS).

'Resource power' is really a subset of position power. Control over the allocation of funds or staff allows you to exert considerable influence in an organisation. Of course, neither of these types of power can be exercised indiscriminately. Our influence is always dependent on the cooperation of others. The ability to withhold collaboration and stop things happening is a form of 'negative power'.

Two further sources of power stem from attributes of individual managers rather than their jobs as such. The authority that is associated with your particular

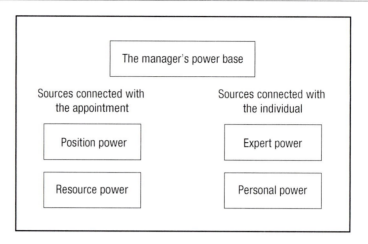

FIGURE 2.1 Sources of power

knowledge rather than your position constitutes 'expert power'. Consultants in the NHS derive considerable power from their specialist expertise. 'Personal power' is what you, personally, bring to the job: style, charisma, the ability to inspire. If your colleagues admire you and respect the way you manage, they will grant you real power as a leader.

STYLE

Classical views of leadership emphasised charisma as personified in an unbroken line of political figures going back before Alexander the Great – Julius Caesar, Napoleon, Hitler, John Kennedy and Nelson Mandela. Military models underline a heroic view of leaders able to inspire devotion and self-sacrifice. Fortunately, a post-heroic view of leadership recognises a more appropriate (and less masculine) set of virtues for the modern health service. Managing subordinates in an appropriate style is more effective than simply commanding or directing them.

How you carry out your managerial functions and the way you exercise power and authority – your management style – is central. To be successful, it must be appropriate to the situation. Different styles are needed at different times and in different organisational contexts. All of us have preferred styles conditioned by personality and experience. The ability to adapt your approach to different circumstances is a major determinant of managerial effectiveness, just as communication skills with individual patients require versatility according to circumstances. Compare your approach to breaking bad news with how you would help a patient stop smoking.

You are likely to have a preferred way of exercising influence. Some people are naturally authoritarian; others more *laissez-faire*. Some managers are dominating; others prefer a more participative approach. Your preferred style is that to which you will naturally default unless you consider that some other style would be more appropriate. This preferred style reflects your own predispositions – your value systems and sense of what is important. How well we tolerate uncertainty is also important. For example, the participative approach involves handing over control to others, with inherent risks. Other important factors include how confident we are in our subordinates, work pressures and stress, which often push people to be more directive.

CONTINGENCY

So how do managers ensure that the management style is appropriate to the circumstances? According to contingency theories of leadership, four variables have to be taken into account when analysing contingent circumstances (unsurprisingly, the one over which you have most control is 'you'!):

1   the manager (or leader) – his or her personality and preferred style
2   the managed (or led) – the needs, attitudes and skills of his or her subordinates or colleagues
3   the task – requirements and goals of the job to be done
4   the context – the organisation and its values and prejudices.

It can be hard to know whether adjustments are needed. Figure 2.2 illustrates the use of a 'best-fit' diagram designed to help decide a management style (on a spectrum from directive to consultative) appropriate to circumstances. Each of the variables will tolerate a small range of styles and the trick is to work out where the overlap occurs. In the hypothetical situation represented here, the organisation dislikes very directive behaviour (context) but the task can be clearly defined. The group doesn't want to be told everything but does not want to be left too much to its own devices and the manager's inclination is towards being a director rather than a democrat.

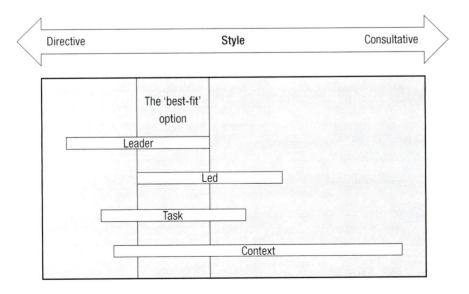

FIGURE 2.2 A 'best-fit' diagram

Plotted like this, the only point where all the requirements overlap is at the consultative end of the manager's range. If he or she is more directive than that, the job will probably get done but in ways that discomfort the group and the organisation.

Fiedler, on the basis of a series of studies, concluded that a more directive style works best in 'situations favourable to the leader' – where the leader is liked and trusted, the task is clearly defined and the leader is powerful in relation to the group.[6] In less favourable circumstances, a supportive, democratic style is more effective. Paradoxically, when circumstances are extremely unfavourable, a directive style may be needed!

Fielder's theory confirms what common sense might suggest: when a task is clearly defined and the leader is clearly in charge, then he or she is expected to get on with the job. In contrast, where a task is ambiguous, where colleagues rather than subordinates are involved and where there is lots of time, all these factors encourage a more cooperative democratic approach. Would Fiedler's recommendations fit comfortably with your preferred style?

There is usually more scope for adjusting contingent circumstances than managers realise. The preferences of colleagues and subordinates (the led) will be

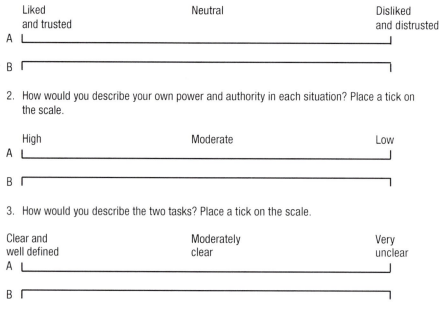

A. Imagine yourself as explaining the layout of a document to your secretary for typing.
B. Imagine yourself as discussing the rearrangement of tasks and rotas in your department with your colleagues and subordinates.

1. How would you describe your credibility in the two situations? Place a tick on the scale.

| Liked and trusted | Neutral | Disliked and distrusted |

2. How would you describe your own power and authority in each situation? Place a tick on the scale.

| High | Moderate | Low |

3. How would you describe the two tasks? Place a tick on the scale.

| Clear and well defined | Moderately clear | Very unclear |

FIGURE 2.3 Using Fiedler's theory to analyse your behaviour in two simple but contrasting situations, A and B

influenced by their expectations of and interest in the particular problem or situation. Their expectations may be shaped by past experience. The nature of the task can be adapted in terms of its complexity and time scales. Even in a modern organisation like the NHS, contextual factors may change. NHS structures alter with each reorganisation and decentralisation may give new project groups new opportunities. Technology is continually evolving, especially in regard to information management.

In summary, the leadership literature is vast. Most textbooks summarise the volume of material by presenting a series of theoretical 'schools' and taxonomies in evolutionary terms.[7] The 'story of leadership' typically opens, as we did, with leader-focused approaches (traits, skills or styles), through situation-based approaches raising the importance of context and contingency, followed by a consideration of the importance of leader–follower relationships, and eventually arriving at transformational approaches concerned with large-scale cultural change. All of these approaches have supplied insights; reflect on them as you observe leaders in your own work setting, for no single theory or model provides an entirely satisfactory explanation of leadership. Kotter notes that 'management is about coping with complexity' whereas 'leadership, by contrast, is about coping with change'.[8] Our view is closer to Mintzberg's – that leadership can be viewed as a subset of management.[9]

KEY POINTS

- A leadership role is inherent in management but there is no single definition of leadership.
- There is a vast literature exploring what makes good leaders; different frameworks can provide you with insights about your own strengths and weaknesses in this role.
- Effective leaders are able to adapt their management styles to varying circumstances – learn from observing others.

REFERENCES

1 Bennis W, Nanus B. *Leaders*. New York: Harper Collins; 1996.
2 Goleman D. *Emotional Intelligence*. London: Bloomsbury Publishing; 1996.
3 Pointer D, Sanchez JP. Leadership in public health practice. In: Scutchfield FD, Keck CW, editors. *Principles of Public Health Practice*. New York: Thomson Delmar Learning; 2003. pp. 140–60.
4 Klein KJ, Ziegert JC, Knight AP, Xiao Y. Dynamic delegation: shared, hierarchical, and deindividualised leadership in extreme action teams. *Adm Sci Q*. 2006; **51**: 590–621.
5 Handy C. *The Age of Unreason*. London: Hutchinson; 1989.
6 Fiedler F. *A Theory of Leadership Effectiveness*. New York: McGraw-Hill; 1967.
7 Northouse P. *Leadership: theory and practice*. London: Sage; 2004.
8 Kotter J. *Leading Change*. Cambridge, MA: Harvard Business School Press; 1996.
9 Mintzberg H. The manager's job: folklore and fact. *Harv Bus Rev*. 1975; **55**: 49–61.

CHAPTER 3

Organisational culture

Q: What do you think is meant by 'organisational culture'?

Culture refers to the ideas and beliefs that give meaning to, but are conceptually separate from, the typical behaviours and structures of a society, community or organisation. Management theorists have borrowed the concept of culture from anthropology.

Different organisations – and parts of organisations – have different cultures. While the culture of the National Health Service (NHS) to an outsider may appear distinctive, different teams, practices or hospitals often have established ways of doing things – a 'different feel'.

Each culture may be more or less appropriate for organisational effectiveness. To operate effectively within an organisation, a manager needs to understand its culture. The concept of culture is fashionable in management circles but needs to be carefully defined. Cultures evolve slowly over time and are influenced by history, ownership, size, technology, objectives, external environment and type of people employed within that organisation.

The key question is whether or not organisational culture is amenable to change. Belief systems and ways in which members of that organisation confer meaning on what they do cannot be easily controlled. For example, attempts to transform the NHS with market-oriented reforms (*see* Section II) have encountered deep-seated cultural resistance. Culture is a matter of beliefs, norms, values and meanings that have been formed over long periods of time. Attitudes to the NHS, among those who use as well as work in it, are deeply held and cannot be changed overnight. They also vary among individuals. To many doctors and managers, for instance, the introduction of 'for-profit' private sector providers is a fundamental challenge to the basic principles of a state-provided NHS. For others, as long as the state funds healthcare free at the point of delivery, private providers are a means of improving NHS care. Changes previously resisted by NHS providers are stimulated when they have to compete to provide a service rather than being the monopoly provider. It is fair to say that, at the first introduction of private providers, the prevalent culture in the NHS resisted reflexly; there is now a more balanced view of its appropriateness. This is an example of culture changing over time through gradual introduction of changing working practices that then become more acceptable.

This is not to say that management should ignore culture and concentrate only on more tangible tasks. Managers can influence an existing culture – through setting an example, through listening to what staff think and feel and offering responses, through their choices of symbolic logos and slogans and through their systems of reward and promotions.

CLASSIFYING CULTURE

The culture of the mammoth teaching hospital is manifestly different from that of general practice, which is different again from that of a mental health trust or a department of social services. They require different kinds of people with different ways of working. There is a growing literature on the culture of organisations, for the customs and traditions of a workplace are a powerful influence on behaviour. Strong abrasive cultures divide organisations into cohesive tribes with distinctively clannish feelings. The values and traditions of the tribe are reinforced by its private language and stories. But not all cultures suit all purposes and people.

A popular early typology described four main types of culture (*see* Figure 3.1).[1]

1 *The power culture* – frequently found in small entrepreneurial organisations in the private sector but could apply to some general practices. Its structure is best pictured as a web. This culture depends on a central power source and places faith in individuals or committees. Such organisations can adapt quickly.

2 *The role culture* – hospitals best fit this model. The accompanying structure can be pictured as a Greek temple. Different clinical teams make up the pillars coordinated at the top by a narrow band of senior doctors and managers, the pediment. Work within and among the pillars is controlled by job descriptions, procedures, guidelines and protocols. Role cultures are often stereotyped as bureaucratic. Role cultures offer security and predictability to the individual. They flourish where economies of scale are more important than flexibility or where technical expertise is more important than product innovation or cost.

3 *The task culture* – job- or project-oriented, this can best be represented structurally as a net. In a so-called 'matrix organisation', much of the power and influence lies in the interstices of the net. The primary care trust or GP consortium with their responsibilities for commissioning different sorts of healthcare could correspond to the task culture. Influence is based more on expert power than position or personal power and this culture is oriented towards teams. It should be able to adapt flexibly to the market or wider environment and it promotes individual autonomy and low status differentials within organisations. Control is retained by the top management allocating projects, people and resources.

4 *The person culture* – the individual is the central focus. There is no structure beyond a cluster of individuals whose purposes such organisations serve. Formerly (one

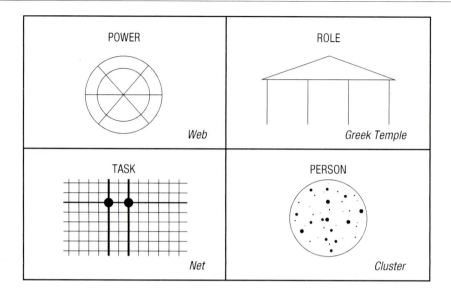

FIGURE 3.1 Culture and structure

hopes), a small general practice or hospital firm led by idiosyncratic doctors might have been described as person cultures. Control mechanisms or management hierarchies are alien to them. Individuals with this orientation are difficult to manage.

Classical management theory was concerned primarily with role cultures and management of the 'steady state'. Modern management thinkers favour the task culture. Journalists and historians, on the other hand, find power cultures centred on key figures more intriguing, while sociologists are concerned with the clash between organisational and individual (person-oriented) values. Other dimensions that have been used to capture the essence of an organisation's culture are shown in Box 3.1.[2]

BOX 3.1 Dimensions of culture (low–high)

1   Innovation and risk taking – degree to which employees are encouraged to be innovative.
2   Outcome orientation – degree to which management focuses on results rather than processes.
3   People orientation – degree to which management decisions consider the effect of outcomes on workers.
4   Team orientation – degree to which activities are organised around teams rather than individuals.
5   Aggressiveness – degree to which people are competitive rather than easy-going.
6   Stability – degree to which organisational activities emphasise the status quo rather than change.

Q: How do you think culture is maintained in an organisation like the NHS?

Mission statements, uniforms and corporate logos as well as building designs provide potent material symbols for reinforcing what Mintzberg calls the 'soul' or culture of any organisation.[3] Edgar Schein suggests that culture is transmitted to organisational members through various forms of socialisation; for example, stories, myths, rituals, rights of passage – and degradation.[4] Humiliation on the ward round or working a 60-hour week provide familiar examples. The so-called 'hidden curriculum', which includes unwritten, taken-for-granted cultural customs and rules for survival, has powerfully shaped the experience of many medical students.[5]

CULTURE IN THE NHS

Research in this area is limited but intriguing. For example, Marshall and colleagues explored the potential tension between the need for managers to produce measurable change and the skills required to produce cultural change and innovation.[6] They used a model called the Competing Values Framework (*see* Figure 3.2), which uses two main dimensions: the first describes how the processes are carried out within the organisation and the second describes the orientation of the organisation to the outside world to generate four basic organisation cultural types. Organisations (or subgroups within them) may possess more than one of these types, but one of them is usually dominant. The framework thus provides a way to describe and explain qualitative information about organisational culture.[7]

Their interviews revealed two distinct and polarised styles of management in primary care trusts. Middle managers tended to interact with doctors in a facilitative way, working with prevailing professional values, while senior managers tended to adopt a more directive style, challenging these values. Much literature in the NHS

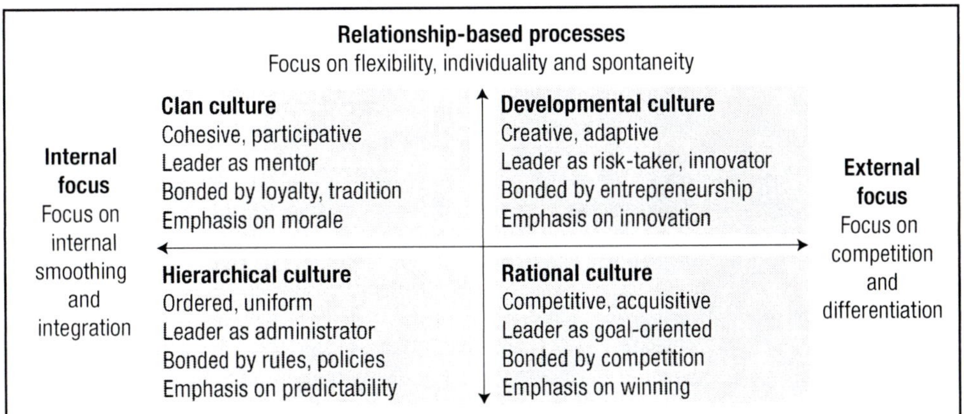

Relationship-based processes
Focus on flexibility, individuality and spontaneity

	Clan culture	Developmental culture	
Internal focus Focus on internal smoothing and integration	Cohesive, participative Leader as mentor Bonded by loyalty, tradition Emphasis on morale	Creative, adaptive Leader as risk-taker, innovator Bonded by entrepreneurship Emphasis on innovation	**External focus** Focus on competition and differentiation
	Hierarchical culture Ordered, uniform Leader as administrator Bonded by rules, policies Emphasis on predictability	**Rational culture** Competitive, acquisitive Leader as goal-oriented Bonded by competition Emphasis on winning	

Mechanistic-type processes
Focus on control, order and stability

FIGURE 3.2 Competing values of organisational cultural types

misleadingly treats managers as if they were a homogenous group. As we have seen, management style is contingent on the roles, responsibilities and the context within which managers work. In particular, senior managers have to reflect the political context within which they work and the policies of the government of the day. They are, however, in a position to exercise significant power and authority, whereas middle managers are more likely to negotiate to achieve their aims.[8] Managers with a directive style are more likely to be promoted within the NHS.

In summary, changing culture to improve quality in a system as complex as the NHS requires a range of different management approaches.[9] A directive, challenging style can, and often does, drive measurable change but may induce some dysfunctional consequences. Managers with a more facilitative style, working with health professionals and retaining their goodwill, while challenging entrenched and outdated practices and cultures, are essential if NHS organisations are to get the best out of the professional workforce. One way of achieving the right balance is to develop healthcare professionals, including doctors, in management and leadership roles. Sustained reform of the NHS is more likely to be achieved if organisations can draw on a repertoire of management styles and leadership skills.

KEY POINTS

- At different stages of your career, you will have you been influenced by your surrounding organisational culture. Use these ways of thinking about culture to describe the team and organisation you work in now.
- The professional cultures of medicine and management can converge or conflict.
- Changing culture to better achieve organisational aims is difficult in a hierarchical monolith like the NHS – but possible!
- Developing health professionals, including doctors, as managers and leaders will benefit the NHS and ultimately patient care.

REFERENCES

1 Handy C. *Understanding Organisations*. 3rd ed. London: Penguin; 1985.
2 Robbins S, Judge T. *Organizational Behaviour*. 12th ed. New Jersey: Prentice Hall; 2007.
3 Mintzberg H, Westley F. Organisational change. *Strategic Management Journal*. 1992; **13**: 39–59.
4 Schein E. *Organisational Psychology*. 3rd ed. London: Prentice Hall; 1980.
5 Lempe H, Seale C. The hidden curriculum in undergraduate medical education: qualitative study of medical students' perceptions of teaching. *BMJ*. 2004; **329**: 770–3.
6 Marshall M, Mannion R, Nelson E, Davies H. Managing change in the culture of general practice: qualitative case studies in primary care trusts. *BMJ*. 2003; **327**: 599–602.
7 Scott J, Mannion R, Davies H, Marshall M. *Organisational Culture and Health Care Performance: a review of the theory, instruments and evidence*. York: Centre for Health Economics, University of York; 2001.

8 Skjorshammer M. Co-operation and conflict in a hospital: interprofessional differences in perception and mangement of conflicts. *J Interprof Care.* 2001; **15**: 7–18.

9 Ferlie EB, Shortell SM. Improving the quality of health care in the United Kingdom and the United States: a framework for change. *Milbank Q.* 2001; **79**: 281–315.

CHAPTER 4

Organisational structure

Q: Can you identify different organisational structures within the NHS?

The term 'organisational structure' refers to the official allocation of tasks and responsibilities to individuals and groups within that organisation. This includes any rules and regulations specifying how relationships between posts and departments should be conducted.

'Centralisation' is the process of concentrating most or all of the organisation's formal authority in one place or in a very limited number of places. If the organisation is strongly hierarchical, centralisation usually takes place at the top of the hierarchy – in the board of directors or chief executive. In a hierarchical organisation, a decentralised authority structure requires delegation to managers or other staff.

'Specialisation' refers to how work is divided up among different individuals or units who can then concentrate on their particular area. As further specialisation proceeds, the greater is the need to coordinate different areas of activity. Larger, more complex organisations like hospitals will develop units specifically devoted to coordination (e.g. clinical directorates or business units).

'Professionalisation' is specialisation of a very particular kind. Hallmarks of professions are monopoly and autonomy.[1] In other words, there is a defined set of activities over which they have a licensed monopoly of practice and within which they have considerable autonomy to operate. A feature of this autonomy has traditionally been self-regulation, the argument being that only those within the profession can understand it; therefore, regulation has to be by the profession of itself.

Health professionals see themselves as accountable in at least four ways: (1) to their peers, (2) to managers where they work, (3) to patients and (4) to their professional body. Health professionals will consider themselves answerable to their professional body (e.g. General Medical Council, Nursing and Midwifery Council) as much as to their employing organisation. Indeed, if their registration with their professional body lapses or is withdrawn they cannot be employed anywhere as a member of that profession. They constitute a distinct type of employee because they have their own source of authority in addition to the usual managerial line of command. This is not usually an issue, since the organisation employs them to deliver services that can only be provided by a member of that profession and, therefore, their professional and managerial accountabilities align. However, management and professional accountabilities can sometimes conflict and may need to be addressed carefully by the professional themselves, their clinical managers and the organisation. If in doubt, the employee should seek professional advice as to the appropriate course of action. For a doctor this would be from their medical director or from the General Medical Council. However, the vast majority of apparent conflicts can be resolved by sensible open discussion between the health professional and their clinical and managerial colleagues. Nowadays, health professionals are increasingly involved in the exercise of public accountability – the obligation placed on public sector organisations to explain and justify their activities to elected representatives or the general public.

One source of variation in the National Health Service (NHS) is the degree to which particular activities are 'formalised'. Thus, while the procedures for purchasing new equipment are usually highly formalised, contracts of employment have been remarkably ill-defined – until recently. Concerns about the vagueness of many doctors' NHS contracts (and therefore how effectively they can be held to account) resulted in their renegotiation in 2004.

Professions ought to encourage the free exchange of ideas and constructive criticism among peers. At best they incorporate ideas on continuing self-improvement and help their members deal with uncertainty and adapt to change. On the other hand, they may encourage a narrow-minded pursuit of self-interest, negative stereotyping of other professions and condescension in dealing with the public. Needless to say, health professionals are an extremely significant feature in the formal structure of the NHS.

Most actual structures, including those in the NHS, reflect a series of compromises or trade-offs. These occur when having more than one desirable characteristic (e.g. public accountability for uniform standards) means having less of another, perhaps equally desirable, characteristic (e.g. decentralisation and local priority setting).

ADMINISTRATION AND BUREAUCRACY

Max Weber famously drew up a list of features of an ideal or pure form of bureaucracy.[2] Studying the development of administration in a diverse range of organisations in Germany, Weber identified the most important characteristics of what he termed 'rational bureaucracy' (*see* Box 4.1). While we sometimes use the term derisively, Weber saw bureaucracy as a powerful replacement for older forms of administration. He did, however, foresee how bureaucracy might intrude into other aspects of human life, eroding the capacity for spontaneous action. One extreme example of controlled management has been termed 'McDonaldisation' – the predictable but dehumanising processes epitomised by chains of fast-food production.[3]

BOX 4.1 Characteristics of Weber's bureaucracy

1 *Specialisation* – the work of individuals and departments is broken down into distinct, routine and well-defined tasks.
2 *Formalisation* – formal rules and procedures are followed to standardise and control the actions of the organisation's members.
3 *Clear hierarchy* – a multilevel 'pyramid of authority' clearly defines how each level supervises the other.
4 *Promotion by merit* – the selection and promotion of staff are based on public criteria (e.g. qualifications or proven competence) rather than on the unexplained preferences of superiors.
5 *Impersonal rewards and sanctions* – rewards and disciplinary procedures are applied impersonally and by standardised procedures.
6 *Career tenure* – job-holders are assured of a job as long as they commit themselves to the organisation.
7 *Separation of careers and private lives* – people are expected to arrange their personal lives so as not to interfere with their activities on behalf of the organisation.

In the language of organisational theorists such as Henry Mintzberg, healthcare organisations are 'professional bureaucracies' rather than 'machine bureaucracies'.[4] One of the characteristics of professional bureaucracies is that front-line staff have a large measure of control over the content of work by virtue of their training and specialist knowledge. Consequently, hierarchical directives issued by those nominally in control often have limited impact and, indeed, may be resisted by front-line staff. In this respect, professional bureaucracies are different from machine bureaucracies (such as government departments). More specifically, they have an inverted power structure in which staff at the bottom of the organisation often have greater influence over decision-making on a day-to-day basis than staff in formal positions of authority. It follows that organisational leaders have to negotiate rather than impose new policies and practices, working in a way that is sensitive to the culture of these organisations.

Control in professional bureaucracies is achieved primarily through horizontal rather than hierarchical processes. These processes are driven by professionals themselves who use collegial influences to secure coordination of work. In healthcare organisations, professional networks play an important role in ensuring control and coordination, both within and among organisations, alongside peer review and peer pressure. Collegial influences depend critically on the credibility of the professionals at their core, rather than simply the power of people in formal positions of authority.

An important feature of professional bureaucracies in Mintzberg's view is that they are oriented to stability rather than change. Not only this but also they are characterised by tribalism and turf wars between professionals who often identify more strongly with 'their' part of the organisation than with the organisation as a whole.

Harrison has defined a dominant form of rationality underpinning contemporary health- and social care policy, which he terms the 'scientific bureaucratic' model.[5] This centres on the assumption that valid and reliable knowledge 'is mainly to be obtained from the accumulation of research conducted by experts according to strict scientific criteria'. Working clinicians are held to be too busy or insufficiently skilled to interpret and apply such knowledge themselves. Professional practice is therefore to be driven by the systematic aggregation and distillation of research findings into protocols, algorithms and guidelines. These are then communicated to practitioners with the expectation that practice will be improved. He argues that this approach is scientific in providing rational foundations for clinical decisions but deficient in taking account of what changes clinical behaviour. The challenge here is to distil research findings into guidelines for best clinical practice – in order to reduce the unwarranted variation that occurs when professionals simply take their own (sometimes idiosyncratic) view on treatments – without undermining professionalism. Medical Royal Colleges and the National Institute for Health and Clinical Excellence (NICE) seek to promote quality improvement and clinical audits while avoiding overly prescriptive protocols that could form the basis of unthinking regulation.

STRUCTURES AND LEADERSHIP

This has several implications for leadership in healthcare.[6] First, in professional bureaucracies, professionals play key leadership roles, both informally and where they are appointed to formal positions. Much more so than in machine bureaucracies, the background of leaders and their standing among peers have a major bearing on their ability to exercise effective leadership, and to bring about change.

Second, professional bureaucracies are characterised by dispersed or distributed leadership. In healthcare organisations, clinical 'microsystems' are a particularly important focus for leadership. It follows that in professional bureaucracies there is a need for large numbers of leaders from clinical backgrounds at different levels. A focus on leadership only at the most senior levels risks missing a central feature of these organisations.

Third, much evidence highlights the importance of collective leadership in healthcare organisations. Collective leadership has two dimensions: first, it refers to the role of leadership teams rather than charismatic individuals; second, it draws attention to the need to bring together constellations of leaders at different levels when major change programmes are undertaken.[7]

Untrammelled medical leadership over the content of work can result in professional bureaucracies becoming anarchic and dysfunctional. Appointing respected and experienced professionals to leadership roles is often advocated as the response to this challenge.[8] However, in itself this may not be sufficient to address the need for control, coordination and innovation. Healthcare organisations have increasingly recognised the requirement to strengthen the role of all staff as followers by investing in organisational development and not just leadership development.

HOW ORGANISATIONAL DESIGN AFFECTS BEHAVIOUR

Alternative organisational designs may better achieve your strategic goals. They can ensure this by promoting more efficient communication and knowledge flows, by strengthening channels of accountability and by motivating organisational members (*see* Chapter 5). Good organisational structure does not by itself produce good performance but a poor organisational structure makes good performance impossible, no matter how good the individual managers may be.[9]

Organisational structures are affected by three particular factors: the environment, technology and size. Some organisations operate in relatively stable environments facing few competitors and limited technological change. In some respects, healthcare delivery, population health needs and what people want from their doctors has not fundamentally altered much in recent decades. For example, wandering around a hospital today, many on sites they have occupied for centuries, our medical forebears would recognise familiar activities. However, in other respects, the business of healthcare (in the literal sense) is changing dramatically.

Considerable evidence shows that organisations operating in uncertain environments are more successful when they adopt structures with organic characteristics; more mechanistic structures suit more predictable environments. Similarly, organisations that employ routine and standardised technologies perform better when structured mechanistically. Smaller firms (fewer than 30 employees) generally have little formal structure. Increasing size means more specialisation, vertical differentiation, more rules and regulations.

> Q: Contrast the size and structure of a typical general practice with a district general hospital.

STRUCTURAL CHANGE

Across the public sector, structural change provides new governments with a beguiling solution to the enduring challenges of cost containment and quality improvement but generally fail to deliver their objectives. There have been at least 15 reorganisations of the NHS in the last three decades. They are frequently cyclical, with ministers hastily reinventing structures that their predecessors had abolished. The associated transition costs are also huge, though often presented as an exercise in cutting bureaucracy. The current Coalition's proposals, which involve abolishing 162 organisations and creating more than 300 new ones, include the implausible claim to be reducing management costs by 45% (*see* Chapter 8). Most important, reorganisations adversely affect service performance during the transition by distracting managers from the real mission of the NHS – to deliver and improve the quality of healthcare.[10] Ideally, such changes should be supported by explicit statements of their measurable costs and benefits, allowing for early analysis of their impact.

> Q: Have you observed productive managerial and clinical time being expended on the current reforms?

In summary, contingency theories as we have seen suggest there is no perfect organisational structure best for all circumstances. Certainly, the NHS is very large and highly diversified and has never been given a single, clear set of goals. There is a wide variety of structures in different parts of the service and considerable tension among goals (e.g. preventing ill health and curing it). Any organisation has both formal and informal sets of relationships and certain patterns of conventional behaviour and expectations. If you want to be effective within your organisation you need to understand its larger structural and cultural dynamics. Analysis of these elements is not an exact science but it can aid you in the workplace. We consider the structure of today's NHS in detail in Section II.

KEY POINTS

- In professional bureaucracies, front-line staff (like doctors) have a large measure of control by virtue of their training and specialist knowledge.
- Consider how the organisational structure within which you work affects your role; how could this be changed to make your team more effective?
- NHS structures have changed with successive reorganisations without realising their intended benefits. Structure should follow function.

REFERENCES

1 Friedson E. Profession of medicine: a study of the sociology of applied knowledge. Chicago: University of Chicago Press; 1970.
2 Weber M. *The Theory of Social and Economic Organization*. London: Collier Macmillan Publishers; 1947.
3 Ritzer G. *The McDonaldization of Society*. 5th ed. Thousand Oaks, CA: Pine Forge Press; 2008.
4 Mintzberg H. *The Structuring of Organisations: a synthesis of the research*. Englewood Cliffs, NJ: Prentice Hall; 1979.
5 Harrison S, Moran M, Wood B. Policy emergence and policy convergence: the case of 'scientific bureaucratic' medicine. *Brit J Polit Int Relat*. 2002; 4: 1–24.
6 Ham C, Dickinson H. *Engaging Doctors in Leadership: what can we learn from international experience and research evidence*. Birmingham: Health Services Management Centre; 2008.
7 Denis J-L, Lamothe L, Langley A. The dynamics of collective leadership and strategic change in pluralistic organisations. *Acad Manage J*. 2001; 44: 809–937.
8 Chantler C. The role and education of doctors in the delivery of health care. *Lancet*. 1999; 353: 1178–81.
9 Drucker P. *Managing for Results*. London: Harper & Row; 1964.
10 Walshe K. Reorganisation of the NHS in England. *BMJ*. 2010; 341: c3843.

CHAPTER 5

Organisational behaviour

Q: What factors affect the behaviour of staff and teams in your workplace?

Organisational behaviour can be studied at three levels: in relation to individuals, in relation to teams and in relation to organisational processes.[1] Managers everywhere are interested in how such concepts as job satisfaction, commitment, motivation and team dynamics may increase productivity, innovation and competitiveness. Having considered organisational structures and cultures, we focus here on individuals and teams.

JOB SATISFACTION

Organisational psychologists identify three components of our attitudes to work: cognitive (what we believe, e.g. my boss treats me unfairly), affective (how we feel, e.g. I dislike my boss) and behavioural (what we are predisposed to do, e.g. I am going to look for another job). Attitudes are important as they influence behaviour.

An early and still widely quoted theory of job satisfaction was elaborated by Herzberg.[2] For Herzberg satisfaction and dissatisfaction were separate dimensions and not opposite sides of the same coin (*see* Figure 5.1). So-called hygiene factors on the left (e.g. the nature of supervision and working conditions) were associated with job dissatisfaction, while motivators on the right (e.g. recognition and responsibility) enhance job satisfaction. The message for managers was that taking care of hygiene factors was a basic prerequisite, a focus on motivating factors would maximise job satisfaction.

In marked contrast, dispositional models of job satisfaction assume it to be a relatively stable characteristic of individuals that changes little in different situations – due to genetic or personality factors. Some long-term studies have indeed found that individuals are consistent in their attitudes to work in different settings. In any event, selecting employees with the 'right attitude' does seem crucial to maintaining a satisfied workforce. Certainly, studies from industry suggest that higher levels of job

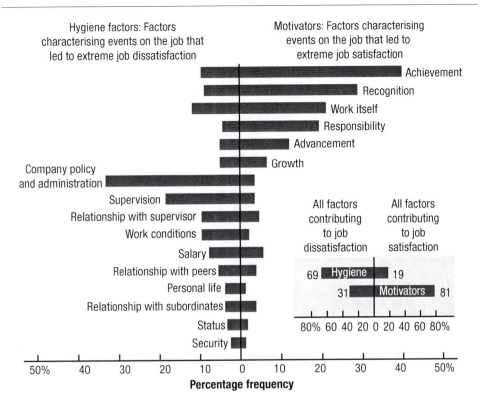

FIGURE 5.1 Theories of job satisfaction – Herzberg's two-factor theory

satisfaction are associated with higher levels of job performance, with lower levels of employee turnover and absenteeism – and more satisfied customers.[3]

One other factor that may influence your job satisfaction is your expectations. This may be relevant in healthcare. For example, negative attitudes among newly qualified doctors may relate to the mismatch between the expectations generated by medical students and the harsh realities of life as a junior doctor.[4]

MOTIVATION

This embraces the psychological forces that determine the direction of people's behaviour, their efforts and level of persistence.[5] Motivation may be extrinsic (tangible rewards) or intrinsic (intangible rewards). While doctors as public servants are well paid, many would argue that the motivating factors in medicine are in large measure intangible – the desire to do good, help others and so forth. Different theories of motivation emphasise different situational factors, including the nature of financial rewards and sanctions, job design and aspects of leadership. There is no single best way of motivating workers but all these factors need to be considered.

The importance of positive reinforcement, setting goals and clarifying expectations is stressed in leadership-based theories. Job enrichment to give more

TABLE 5.1 David McClelland's needs theory

Need for achievement	The need to accomplish goals, excel and strive continually to do things better
Need for power	The need to influence and lead others, and be in control of one's environment
Need for affiliation	The desire for close and friendly interpersonal relationships

control over content, planning and execution can help motivate employees. David McClelland considered the importance of matching people and job-related rewards, recognising three different sorts of personal need (*see* Table 5.1).[6]

> **Q:** How much do you think you will need achievement, power and affiliation in your future work?

WORKING IN TEAMS

It is a truism to say that much healthcare is delivered through multidisciplinary teams and understanding how teams work and how you can make them effective is universally agreed to be a core attribute of the good doctor.[7] Ironically, for many older doctors, the best example of a functional team was the clinical 'firm'. Increasingly, with the advent of the European Working Time Directive and moves to shift work, such firms no longer exist. The team can be defined as a group whose members have complementary skills and common goals for which they hold themselves mutually accountable.

Central to your effectiveness in teams is an understanding of your role (*see* Box 5.1). However, our view of how we are supposed to act in a given situation may not be shared by others. Uncertainty or divergent expectations about one's role can be a major source of job-related stress.

BOX 5.1 Aspects of role

- *Role* – a set of typical behaviour patterns attributed to someone occupying a given position
- *Role perception* – our view of how we're supposed to act in a given situation
- *Role expectation* – others' views of how we're supposed to act in a given situation
- *Role conflict* – divergent role expectations
- *Role ambiguity* – uncertainty about one's role

Norms or the informal rules that guide team members' behaviour are another important influence on team working. Norms relate not just to how team members should perform but also how they relate to one another or even to how they dress! (*See* Box 5.2.)

BOX 5.2 Norms

- *Norms* – generally agreed-upon informal rules that guide group members' behaviour (prescriptive or prospective)
- *Performance norms* – explicit cues on how hard members should work and how to approach particular tasks
- *Allocation of resources norms* – influence work allocation, distribution of equipment, perks
- *Social arrangement norms* – regulate social interactions within the group (e.g. level of deference, friendship inside and outside the group)
- *Appearance norms* – e.g. appropriate dress and demeanour

Roles and norms in turn relate to the status accorded to teams or individual team members by others. This is determined by the power a person wields over others (*see* Chapter 2), how that person contributes to group goals and his/her personal characteristics. High-status members are often more assertive, given more freedom to deviate from group norms and are less likely to conform to group expectations. The National Health Service (NHS) is notoriously hierarchical and status differentials can create internal tensions.

Q: Have you encountered any 'difficult' colleagues? Why might they have been difficult to manage?

The cohesiveness of teams – the degree to which team members share common attitudes, values and identity – is a further factor tending to increase output, at least where performance norms are strong. Team cohesiveness increases when members spend time together, as group size decreases, with success in achieving goals – and where there is a common 'enemy' (like 'management'!).

Q: List the teams in which you work. Think about your own role within these teams. Do your perceptions of the role differ from the expectations of others? Can you think of any conflicts or ambiguity relating to your role?

Several writers have related group tensions to productivity and described stages in the development of any team. One such model is shown in Figure 5.2.[8]

Q: Looking back on your experiences in particular teams, can you relate to any of these stages?

Ultimately, what matters from a managerial perspective is the team's effectiveness. This is influenced by a constellation of factors including team composition, how work is designed and contextual factors such as the availability of adequate resources and clear leadership (*see* Chapter 13).

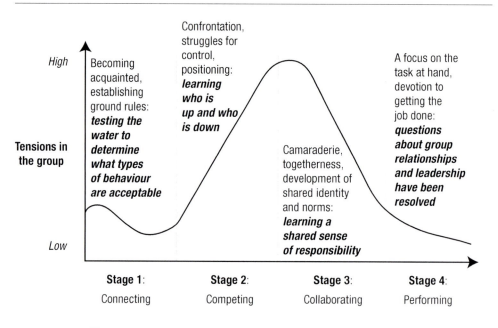

FIGURE 5.2 The stages of team development

In conclusion, membership of groups and teams has a powerful effect on individual behaviour. We are all aware that social dynamics can create performance problems but teams have an enormous potential to improve performance through their distinctive architecture (roles, norms and status, etc.) In particular, building or leading an effective team requires careful management of the tension between individual diversity and conformity to group processes and goals. Developing appropriate structures and roles plays a key part in addressing this tension.

CHANGING ORGANISATIONAL BEHAVIOUR

Q: Looking back over what we have covered so far, what sort of changes do you think have to be managed in organisations like the NHS? We have already touched on five sorts of change:
1   strategic change
2   structural change
3   financial change
4   changes to work processes
5   cultural change.

Various models have been proposed to help manage change. One of the best known, formulated by John Kotter, is used below.[9] Another time-honoured framework for thinking about organisational change is associated with Kurt Lewin.[10] He described three stages in the evolution of organisational change (*see* Figure 5.3). The first

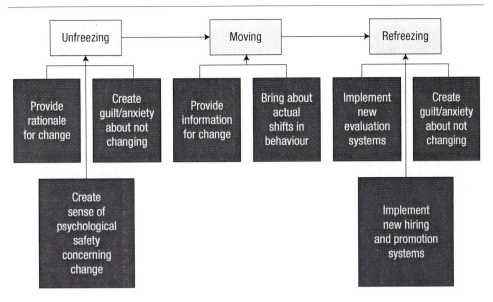

FIGURE 5.3 Kurt Lewin's model of planned change

involves 'unfreezing' established processes and practices; the second involves moving these same things, change itself; the third he termed 'refreezing', bedding down these changes. Lewin's model helps to remind us that change can be mismanaged. If processes are refrozen in the wrong place or resistance to change deepens as a consequence, change can be actively harmful.

Proposed change is always more appealing to some group members than others and will meet some resistance accordingly. Whether or not change occurs comes down ultimately to whether its perceived 'cost' (in the broader sense) outweighs its benefits, as well as to levels of dissatisfaction with the status quo (*see* Box 5.3).

BOX 5.3 Establishing the need for change (after Beckhard and Gleicher)

$C = [A \times B \times D] > X$ where:

C = Change
A = Level of dissatisfaction with the status quo
B = Desirability of the proposed change or end state
D = Perceived feasibility of the change
X = Perceived 'cost' of changing

Over the last few years, dialogues within the NHS seem to have been drowned out by the rhetoric of change. In the face of economic constraints, this is understandable. In order to deliver the same amount of care in the face of increasing need and demand and within finite budgets, new ways of delivering care (often termed 'innovation') are required. Finding new ways of working is important but such change may, nevertheless, meet with resistance at three levels.

1 *Organisational* – hierarchical, mechanistic structures dominated by professional interests battling for power and control over resources will be more resistant to change.

2 *Group* – strongly cohesive teams reinforcing norms and roles will be harder to change.

3 *Individual* – natural insecurity, mistrust based on past experience and a tendency to protect material interests will all impede change.

> **Q:** Thinking about changes you have experienced at work, can you think of ways in which individuals expressed support or resistance?

Table 5.2 lists different ways of expressing resistance to change with which you will already be familiar. Watch out for others!

TABLE 5.2 Expressions of resistance

Positive	Negative
Open-minded questioning	Not coming to meetings
Disagreeing with the rationale of the change	Being too busy to attend training
Lobbying for alternative solutions	Pulling people out of workshops
Analysing and appraising alternatives	Starting with another initiative

---

KEY POINTS

- An understanding of the factors affecting work behaviour of individuals and teams is central to effective management.
- Consider the factors that satisfy and motivate you in the workplace.
- Attempts to reform the NHS often founder for lack of understanding of the factors that shape professional behaviour.

REFERENCES

1 Greenberg J, Baron R. *Behaviour in Organisations: understanding and managing the human side of work.* 2nd ed. Boston: Allyn & Bacon; 1990.

2 Herzberg F. *Work and the Nature of Man.* Cleveland: World Publishing Company; 1966.

3 Robbins S, Judge T. *Organizational Behaviour.* 12th ed. New Jersey: Prentice Hall; 2007.

4 Goldacre M, Lambert T, Evans J, Turner G. Preregistration house officers' views on whether their experience at medical school prepared them well for their jobs: national questionnaire survey. *BMJ.* 2003; **326**: 1011–12.

5 Shah J, Gardner W, editors. *Handbook of Motivation Science*. New York: Guilford Press; 2008.

6 McClelland D. *Human Motivation*. New Jersey: General Learning Press; 1973.

7 General Medical Council. *Tomorrow's Doctors: outcomes and standards for undergraduate medical education*. London: GMC; 2009.

8 Gadon H, Josefowitz N, editors. *Fitting In: how to get a good start in your new job*. Reading, MA: Addison-Wesley; 1988.

9 Kotter J. *Leading Change*. Cambridge, MA: Harvard Business School Press; 1996.

10 Lewin K. Frontiers of group dynamics. *Hum Relat*. 1947; **1**: 5–41.

CHAPTER 6

Health policy

Q: What do you know about health policy and how it affects you?

An understanding of how policy is made is an important means by which medical practitioners can comprehend the service within which they work – and perhaps change it. The policy process is the means by which particular policies emerge and are pursued by governments and government agencies. Policy is best understood as the consequence of the interrelation of 'actors' (those people or organisations populating the process), the wider context, the process by which policy is made and the content of the policy itself (i.e. what it is designed to achieve).[1] (*See* Figure 6.1.)

WHAT DO WE MEAN BY POLICY?

A common-sense approach would equate public policy with the formal decisions or explicit proposals of governments or public agencies. In practice, the process of

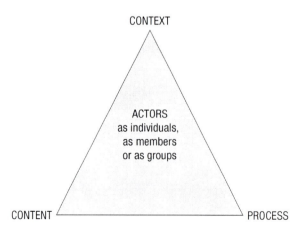

FIGURE 6.1 Walt–Gibson model for policy analysis

policymaking is subtler. Policy may emerge from a series of apparently unrelated decisions and governments or public agencies do not control the outcomes of intended policies with any great certainty. In fact, government policy may be as much about what they choose not to do as about what they choose to do.[2]

> Q: Can you think of any unexpected consequences of recent governments' health policies?

Descriptions of the policy process as a system have been dominated in recent years by two opposing schools of thought – the 'rationalists' and the 'incrementalists'. 'Rational' models of the policy process describe it in terms of a series of linked, but distinct, phases and types of activity that together produce 'a policy'. Such an approach is based on the application of a logical and apparently sequential set of functions and technical skills to ensure that an appropriate response is generated to a 'policy problem'. For example, Walt and Gilson describe four key stages: (1) problem identification and issue recognition, (2) policy formulation, (3) policy implementation and (4) policy evaluation.[1]

While such a rational model is attractive, Lindblom has criticised the notion that values and objectives (i.e. the policy 'ends') can be identified separately to any consideration of the policy 'means'.[3] In actual decision-making, he suggested, policymakers should not set prior aims but should seek only to move from the status quo by small steps and by reaching agreement among competing interest groups – human beings simply do not possess the ability to process all necessary information to make 'rational' decisions.

THE CONTEXT FOR POLICYMAKING

Policies exist in a 'context' that reflects both constraints and opportunities within the broader environment within which any policy is located. Leichter identified four distinct sets of contextual factors that would impact on national health policy: (1) situational factors (transient conditions such as war that allow governments to introduce policies otherwise considered out of bounds), (2) structural factors (relatively unchanging elements in society such as the political regime), (3) cultural factors (reflecting the values within society) and (4) environmental factors (those that impinge on states from their contact with other countries).[4] At a more practical level, context will include factors such as the existing relationships among organisations, local interest groups and the population's health status.

One important contextual factor of particular interest to students of health policy is that of 'professionalism'. As we have seen, professionals wield power by virtue of their specialist knowledge, ability to control the supply of their membership and to regulate their own affairs. As a result professionals enjoy high degrees of autonomy and discretion.

Alford's classic study of the New York health system identified key interests within the policy process.[5] 'Professional monopolisers' (the medical profession) were the dominant power, challenged only by 'corporate rationalisers' (managerial interests) who sought to exert control over the medical professionals. The interests of community groups and patients exercised little power within the healthcare system and were described by Alford as 'repressed'. Importantly, Alford suggested that professional power allowed the medical interest group to control the ideological and cultural environment that supported their dominant position.

The position of the medical profession within the British policy process has been described as a 'state-licensed elite'. The predominance of medical interests since the formation of the National Health Service (NHS) has been held to represent a form of 'ideological corporatism', where governments and the profession share a similar world view.[6] However, a number of conflicts emerged between government and the medical profession. For example, the introduction of market-based reforms to the NHS since the 1980s has been a source of ongoing dispute between government and the British Medical Association. Successive governments have also changed the contractual terms that bound both independently contracted and employed professionals to the NHS. The fact that many of these reforms were pursued in the teeth of opposition from professional interests suggests that the prevailing corporatist accommodation between government and professions is weaker now than it once was.[7]

IMPLEMENTATION AS PART OF THE POLICY PROCESS

In the rational models of the policy process described, implementation features as a distinct phase that occurs once the formal 'policy' has been created. Implementation is seen as simply a 'technical' or 'managerial' process, unconnected to the more vital issue of policy content.

This 'top-down' conceptualisation of the policy process (where managers faithfully implement policy coming down from a political policymaking cadre) has been challenged by a welter of empirical studies. These studies suggest that policy implementation is fundamentally intertwined with policymaking. In this view, policy is made 'bottom-up' by those responsible for implementation.[8]

The bottom-up approach is based on two propositions: that the selection of policy solutions may occur during implementation (i.e. policies may not always be clearly defined prior to their operationalisation) and that the behaviour of implementers may mediate the policy content or its outcome. For example, Lipsky identified a key role for 'street-level bureaucrats' who were able to alter policy outcomes through the way in which they chose to respond to pressures from above.[9] An examination of Dutch policy on heart transplants showed that national policy was deliberately subverted by health service providers.[10]

Healthcare institutions therefore may pursue their own organisational strategies and policymaking agenda and are unlikely to see themselves as passive implementers of government policy. Indeed, NHS organisations have their own collective interest group (the NHS Confederation) that actively promotes policy and seeks to influence government opinion. All this means that ministers' ability to achieve change on the ground is rather more constrained than they might wish.

Finally, doctors influence policy both collectively – via their trade union, the British Medical Association – and individually. Think of the recent contribution of Lord Ara Darzi, a surgeon at St Mary's Hospital.[11] Politicians are all too aware of the power of a profession that makes contact with six million people a week!

RECENT HEALTH POLICY

This section considers briefly some of the main features of health policy in England since the election of the Labour government in 1997. Note that in post-devolution-era England, Wales and Scotland have adopted very different health policies. However, the substance of all major policy documents and White Papers in recent decades can be summarised in terms of a few central themes (*see* Box 6.1).

BOX 6.1 Common policy concerns

- Cost containment and efficiency
- Improving access
- Variations in quality of care
- Increasing user involvement/choice
- Info management/technology
- Equity
- Workforce development

The Labour government's reforms comprised three overlapping strategies.[12] The first dimension of reform was to improve the provision of care through a mix of initiatives such as increasing the supply of professionals, supporting learning and innovation and improving the physical infrastructure. This was supported by a major leap in NHS funding announced in 2000. Current commitments to NHS spending increases suggest that UK spending on health (both public and private) rose from around 7% of gross domestic product (GDP) in 2000 to about 10% in 2010, a proportion of GDP approaching that of the European average.

The second dimension of reform involved setting national standards and targets, introducing inspection of providers, intervening in local provision where required and publishing information on performance. The third dimension of reform involved the development of the commissioning function in local health agencies, giving patients the right to choose their provider and introducing a diverse market of providers supported by new financial incentives.

Labour's approach to health policy relied on both top-down and highly directive central planning while simultaneously creating a mechanism designed to drive change from the bottom up. Moreover, a new political consensus around the management of the NHS emerged – at the 2005 and 2010 general elections the similarities between the major political parties in terms of their plans for the NHS was startling.

MARKETS: THE DRIVE FOR EFFICIENCY AND COST CONTAINMENT

The Labour Party came to power in 1997 advocating an end to competitive markets and private sector involvement in clinical services, promoting instead a more cooperative planning approach. An early, and highly symbolic, act was to abolish GP fundholding (where general practitioners received budgets with which to purchase some of their patients' care).

Yet the main architecture of the quasi-market was retained – notably the split between purchasing and providing – and, ultimately, the Labour governments went further in introducing market-inspired reforms than their Conservative predecessors would have dared. The main features of this market-based system included:

➤ new financial incentives (fees for each treatment given) designed to promote competition among providers
➤ rights for patients to choose their providers
➤ diversification of supply in hospital and primary care to include the independent sector
➤ greater autonomy of NHS providers through the replacement of central accountability of NHS hospitals to the Department of Health with accountability of 'foundation trusts' to local people and to an independent regulator.

The Coalition government is building on these developments as we will see in Chapter 8.

So what explained the move towards markets?[13] First, the substantial investment in NHS services since 2000 saw productivity fall, at least as measured by the NHS 'efficiency index' (put simply, rises in clinical activity did not match the rises in funding). There was concern that an abundance of funds had led to inefficient practices and only modest gains for patients. There was a parallel concern that the public monopoly nature of the NHS had also led to a lack of responsiveness to the needs of individual patients. Without challenge, and the potential for patients to 'exit' the system, providers may lack motivation to listen to their customers. Policies that promoted 'patient choice', underpinned by financial incentives rewarding hospitals that attract more custom, were intended to improve responsiveness to the needs of patients.

BETTER HEALTH AS WELL AS BETTER HEALTH SERVICES?

While much of the public's attention has been drawn towards the debate over how best to improve health services, the Labour government of 1997 to 2010 also developed a substantial public health agenda (*see* Box 6.2). The financial as well as health benefits of securing a healthier population were described by Sir Derek Wanless.[14] In his projection of health expenditure, Wanless calculated that healthcare for a population that was not involved in promoting its own health would be significantly more expensive than one that was 'fully engaged'. The government claimed some success: targets for reduced deaths from cancer and heart disease look set to be met. Yet, when looked at more critically, many of the achievements are simply in line with longer-term trends in disease prevention and survival.

BOX 6.2 Government priorities for public health

Priorities for action in *Choosing Health: making healthy choices easier.*[15]
- reducing the number of people who smoke
- reducing obesity and improving diet and nutrition
- increasing exercise
- encouraging and supporting sensible drinking
- improving sexual health
- improving mental health.

A further area of commitment is to reduce inequalities in health between the richest and poorest populations. Policies addressing the social determinants of health require working across many sectors (health, education, criminal justice, local government, transport, etc.) and more effective interdepartmental working. This requires what is often referred to as a 'whole systems approach' (although it is not always clear what this means in practice). Commonly understood characteristics of whole systems working include:

➤ that services are responsible to the needs of individual patients/clients
➤ that all stakeholders accept their interdependency
➤ that partnerships are advanced by sharing a vision of the service priorities
➤ that users of the system do not experience unnecessary gaps or duplication.

A key target for 2010 was to reduce by at least 10% the gap between the fifth of local authority areas with the lowest life expectancy at birth and the population as a whole. A succession of reviews examined health inequalities but evidence so far suggests that health inequalities are continuing to widen.[16] The Coalition government from 2010 has stated a commitment to reduce inequalities, and has made implementation of the Marmot review of health inequalities, commissioned by the previous Labour administration, a part of its public health policy.[17]

In summary, the NHS in England underwent significant change under the Labour government. It showed a clear preference for market incentives over central planning but these policy solutions had little effect on the familiar problems that they were designed to address: rising demand and indifferent productivity. On the left of the political spectrum, commentators hold this up as evidence that 'markets don't work';[18] those to the right claim that this illustrates the need to strengthen market mechanisms and the role of private providers. As we will see in the next section, the incoming Coalition government has pledged another major overhaul of the NHS. Despite evidence for the limited impact of previous reorganisations, they look set to restore something akin to the fundholding model dismantled by their predecessors. This well illustrates the cyclical nature of much policymaking, based as it is more on ideology than evidence.

KEY POINTS

- Rational models of planning and policymaking underplay the contingent, ad hoc nature of these processes in practice.
- Policymaking is a political process and only ever partially evidence-based.
- Understanding how policy is made can help you influence its development and implementation locally.

REFERENCES

1 Walt G and Gilson L. *Health Policy: an introduction to process and power.* London: Zed Books; 1994.
2 Dye T. *Top Down Policymaking.* London: Chatham House Publishers; 2001.
3 Lindblom CE 1959, The science of muddling through. *Public Admin Rev.* 2001; **19**: 79–88.
4 Leichter HM. *A Comparative Approach to Policy Analysis: healthcare policy in four nations.* Cambridge: Cambridge University Press; 1979.
5 Alford RR. *Healthcare Politics.* Chicago: University of Chicago Press; 1975.
6 Dunleavy P. Professions and policy change: notes towards a model of ideological corporatism. *Public Administration Bulletin.* 1981: **36**; 3–16.
7 Klein R. *The New Politics of the NHS.* 3rd ed. London: Longman; 1995.
8 Lewis R. Health policy. In: Gillam S, Yates J, Badrinath P, editors. *Essential Health: policy and practice.* Cambridge: Cambridge University Press; 2007. pp. 257–70.
9 Lipsky M. Towards a theory of street-level bureaucracy. In: Hawley WD, editor. *Theoretical Perspectives on Urban Politics.* Englewood Cliffs, NJ: Prentice-Hall; 1976. pp. 196–213.
10 De Roo A, Maarse H. Understanding the central-local relationship in health care: a new approach. *Int J Health Plann Manage.* 1990; **5**: 15–25.
11 Darzi A. Quality and the NHS next stage review. *Lancet.* 2008; **371**: 1563–4.
12 Stevens S. Reform strategies for the English NHS. *Health Aff.* 2004; **23**(3): 37–44.
13 Lewis R and Dixon J. *NHS Market Futures: exploring the impact of health service market reforms.* London: The King's Fund; 2005.
14 Wanless D. *Securing Our Future Health: taking a long-term view.* Final report. London: HM Treasury; 2002.
15 Department of Health. *Choosing Health: making healthy choices easier.* London: The Stationery Office; 2004.
16 Department of Health. *Healthy Lives, Healthy People: our strategy for public health in England.* London: The Stationery Office; 2010.
17 Marmot M. Strategic review of health inequalities in England post-2010. Marmot review final report. University College London; 2010. Available at: www.ucl.ac.uk/gheg/marmotreview/Documents (accessed 21 January 2011)
18 Pollock A. *NHS plc: the privatisation of our health care.* London: Verso; 2004.

Management and leadership in practice

CHAPTER 7

Historical perspectives

Q: How has the relationship between managers and doctors changed since 1948?

Doctors have traditionally enjoyed much freedom to practise in the way they consider appropriate. At the inception of the National Health Service (NHS) in 1948, the government provided a framework within which the health professions could provide treatment and care for patients according to their own independent professional judgement of patients' needs. This independence remains a central feature in the management of health services. Hospital consultants' clinical autonomy derived from what was, in effect, a bargain between the state and the medical profession whereby 'central government controlled the budget, while doctors controlled what happened within that budget. Financial power was concentrated at the centre; clinical power was concentrated at the periphery'.[1]

In the early years of the NHS, managers or administrators were appointed 'to provide and organise the facilities and resources for professionals to get on with their work'.[2] Administrators were not the driving forces in their authorities but tended to act as specific problem-solvers rather than in pursuit of defined objectives – to be reactive. Other groups of employees were the focus of their work rather than users of the health service. Maintaining existing health services was central, with planning being conceived mainly in terms of small, ad hoc, incremental improvements. The status quo was seldom subject to critical scrutiny. The role of the 'manager as diplomat' was symbolised by the official policy of so-called consensus management.

Growing financial pressures in the NHS during the 1970s and 1980s led to a realignment of the relationship between managers, on the one hand, and doctors and other health professions, on the other. A generally accepted landmark is the report of the Griffiths inquiry into NHS management (1985), chaired by the chair of Sainsbury's. This argued for a system of general management to be introduced in place of so-called consensus management – to provide the NHS with effective leadership and to ensure clear accountability for decision-making.[3]

The Griffiths report also argued that hospital doctors 'must accept the management responsibility which goes with clinical freedom'. Most NHS hospitals implemented a system of medical management centred on the appointment of senior doctors as clinical directors responsible for leading the work of different services within the hospital. Clinical directors combine their management and leadership roles with continuing but reduced clinical duties. They usually work with a nurse manager and a business manager in a management triumvirate. Clinical directors often come together as a group with the medical director and chief executive to advise on developments across the hospital as a whole.

While doctors took on more non-clinical responsibilities, managers were increasingly involved in questioning medical priorities. However, any shift in the balance of power between managers and doctors was limited and the dominance of the medical profession remained largely intact.[4] This perception was reinforced by the events leading up to the failures in paediatric heart surgery at Bristol described in the Introduction, where the prevailing culture emphasised the importance of clinical autonomy.

The internal market inaugurated by a Conservative government in the early 1990s extended the management responsibilities of general practitioners too. They were given budgets with which to purchase secondary care for their patients. Fundholding capitalised on their knowledge of local services and financial entrepreneurialism to drive efficiencies although the evidence for its impact is disputed.[5]

PLUS ÇA CHANGE?

Ironically, attempts to change the management culture within the NHS have often illustrated the immutability of prevailing norms. Various factors have inhibited cultural change; in particular, the continuing lack of a single set of clear managerial objectives. The task culture is project-oriented but what project is the NHS engaged in? Care, cure or prevention? Managers were given no fresh powers with which to redress their relationship with the medical profession, which frequently behaved as bearers of a different, rival culture. The last decade has, at least, provided additional resources with greater scope for innovation.

Did the Griffiths report implant a new management culture in the NHS? Most of the early research identified only limited changes. Twenty years on, rather more has changed. We have seen the advent of more flexible organisational structures: integrated care organisations, foundation trusts, practice-based commissioning consortia and the rest. The majority of health professionals work constructively alongside managerial colleagues and many play important leadership roles. A much greater focus on users' priorities – as reflected in an acceptance of waiting time targets, booking choices, and responsiveness to the views of patients – is evident. Altogether, managers are impressively responsive to central policy dictates, although the limitations of a target-driven culture in the NHS are widely acknowledged. (There are benefits too.)

In summary, the Griffiths reforms are best seen as the start of a long-term process of renegotiating the role of the medical profession in the NHS. This process continued with the introduction of market-oriented organisational reforms during the 1990s and beyond. However, established relationships of power and influence in the NHS have proved surprisingly durable. Attempts to make the NHS more 'businesslike' and to bridge the divide between managers and doctors are ongoing.

CONTEMPORARY CHALLENGES

In recent years, NHS leaders have tended to hit the headlines for the wrong reasons. Recurring themes are media outrage about senior pay, allegations of too many managers and the perceived role of NHS leaders in failing to resolve major incidents.

However, both common sense and the research evidence tell us that these accusations are unfair. In the current financial climate, our previous faith as a society in private sector models of financing has been significantly dented. In reality, the track record of public service leaders as good stewards of public resources looks even more impressive. An organisation as large and complex as the NHS requires all the management and leadership it can get, and needs the best skills available to be successful.

While important, leadership is only one of a number of factors that shape a service or an organisation and how it performs. The work of James Reason and others suggest that responses to adverse events can adopt a *person approach* (blaming individuals for perceived mistakes) or a *systems approach* (which sees poor practice as the result of the conditions under which people work and the way the system is organised). When major incidents occur, it is tempting to blame *active failures* by individual workers or leaders, yet probably more fruitful to focus on the *latent conditions* (the underlying context that enabled such events to occur in the first place).[6]

If the success of healthcare systems were judged according to the size of the organisation and the number of people it treats, the NHS would be towards the top of the league table as one of the largest organisations in the world treating over one million people every 36 hours.[7] Over time the NHS has grown in both size and complexity; consequently, the role of management has needed to change in order to keep pace with this rapid development. Yet despite experiencing unprecedented levels of funding and having managed to reduce outpatient waiting times, the NHS still ranks behind other European countries in health outcomes and recent hospital scandals seem to demonstrate potential weaknesses in leadership and management practices. While well-managed services and high-quality leadership can lead to better outcomes for patients,[8] a major challenge for the NHS remains ensuring it has high-quality leadership at all levels of the organisation.

REFERENCES

1 Klein R. *The New Politics of the NHS.* 5th ed. Oxford: Radcliffe Publishing; 2006.

2 Harrison S, Pollitt C. *Controlling the Health Professionals: the future of work and organization in the NHS.* Buckingham: Open University Press; 1994.

3 Griffiths Report. NHS Management Inquiry. HMSO: London; 1995.

4 Ham C, Dickinson H. *Engaging Doctors in Leadership: what can we learn from international*

experience and research evidence. Birmingham: Health Services Management Centre; 2008.

5 Le Grand J, Mays N, Mulligan J. *Learning from the NHS Internal Market: a review of the evidence.* London: The King's Fund; 1998.

6 Reason J. Human error: models and management. *BMJ.* 2000; **320**: 768–70.

7 NHS Confederation. NHS Choices empowering patients through information. Briefing 145. London; 2007.

8 Firth Cozens J, Mowbray D. Leadership and the quality of care. *Qual Health Care.* 2001; 10: ii3-ii7 doi: 10.1136/qhc.0100003.

CHAPTER 8

The NHS: structure and functions

with Paul Cosford

Q: What kind of organisational structure does the National Health Service (NHS) have? How centralised is the NHS? How formalised are its procedures and ways of working? How would you describe the lines of command?

In recent years, two opposing tendencies have been much in evidence. On the one hand, health professionals such as GPs and consultants have had plenty of freedom to organise themselves as they see fit, while health authorities have also varied greatly in their detailed organisational structures. On the other hand, the introduction of general management has strengthened line management, demanding more detailed regulation about the delivery of health services. The approach of recent Labour governments has been to set national targets for the NHS to deliver locally, which has strengthened this trend. The Coalition government has a contrasting approach. This is to focus on delegating power and responsibility to a local level, such as to groups of practices commissioning NHS care, with a requirement to improve the outcomes of healthcare. The intention is to focus on outcomes of care that are particularly important to local people.

This chapter examines how the NHS works, borrowing from an excellent junior doctors' guide to the NHS.[1] The key organisations in respect of the NHS are:
- parliament
- the Department of Health
- commissioners – organisations that commission care on behalf of the community they serve (currently primary care trusts)
- providers – organisations that provide care
- so-called 'arm's-length bodies' with a variety of functions including protecting the public's health (the Health Protection Agency), regulating healthcare providers (Monitor), setting standards for NHS provision (National Institute for Health and Clinical Excellence (NICE)), and others
- intermediate-tier organisations (currently strategic health authorities), which

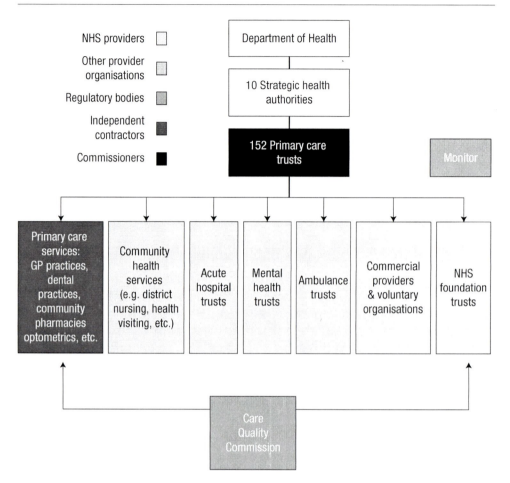

FIGURE 8.1 Current structure of the NHS

> support, coordinate and ensure the performance of the complex healthcare system at a regional level
> ➤ local authorities, which also have many closely related functions such as public health, social care and children's services.

PARLIAMENT

Parliament is responsible for approving legislation and forming the framework in which the health service operates. Parliament determines the budget to be spent on health and healthcare, and holds the Department of Health to account for its spending of taxpayers' money and operation of the National Health Service. The amount of resource parliament decides to spend on healthcare is historically prioritised over most other calls on public expenditure. From 2002/03 to 2007/08 there was an annual increase of 10% year on year in the money provided to the Department of Health, much more than for other public services such as education and criminal justice. Similarly, the Coalition government has committed to maintain health spending while reducing spend in other public services.

THE DEPARTMENT OF HEALTH

The Department of Health (DH) is a government department, headed by the Secretary of State for Health. It is based in London and Leeds and is accountable to the public through parliament. The DH does not directly deliver health or social care services to the public; it works with delivery partners, including the NHS, local government and arm's-length bodies. The latter have a role in the process of national government, but are not part of government departments. They operate at arm's length from ministers. They are sponsored by government departments and derive all or part of their funding from their sponsor departments. The DH's goals are twofold:

1   attainment of better health, well-being, care and value for the country
2   provision of leadership for the NHS, social care and public health.

The DH does this in the following ways.

➤ *Setting direction for the NHS, adult social care, and public health* – policy, strategy, legislation, resource allocation, and an NHS operating framework that sets out the priorities for the NHS each year.
➤ *Supporting delivery of care* – performance monitoring, managerial leadership, building capacity and capability and ensuring value for money.
➤ *Leading health and well-being on behalf of the government* – working with other government departments, third and private sectors and international partners.
➤ *Accounting to parliament and the public* – answering parliamentary questions and communicating to the public via the media, letters, visits and speeches.

Three people are responsible for managing the DH.

1   *Permanent Secretary* – a senior civil servant responsible for overall leadership and management of the DH, ensuring that it operates efficiently and coherently as a department of state in support of ministers.
2   *Chief Medical Officer* – the government's chief adviser on medical issues and public health.
3   *NHS Chief Executive* – the government's chief adviser on NHS issues and leader of the NHS.

The Coalition government is currently separating the Department of Health's functions into two distinct elements (*see* Figure 8.2).

➤ The *NHS Commissioning Board*, which will manage the NHS in England, and will effectively be separate from the DH. The aim is to reduce political control (and 'interference') over the management of the NHS.
➤ The *Public Health Service*, which will provide national policy leadership for improving health and will deliver the health protection services currently provided by the Health Protection Agency among others.

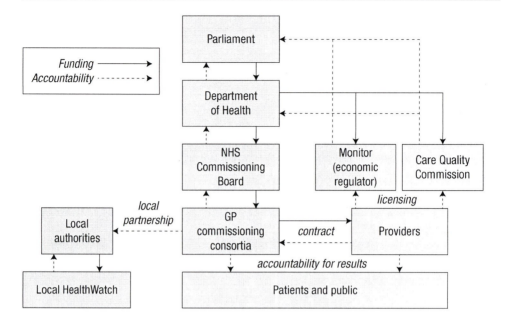

FIGURE 8.2 Future structure of the NHS

COMMISSIONING

The majority of healthcare is currently commissioned by primary care trusts (PCTs), which place contracts with providers of NHS care (such as acute hospital trusts). The commissioning of healthcare will transfer to GP commissioning groups ('clusters') in 2012 under the current plans of the Coalition government.[2]

Commissioning is the process of determining the health needs of the population, the resources available and how to organise service provision. Commissioning occurs mainly at PCT level following a joint strategic needs assessment (JSNA) conducted in partnership by local government, PCTs and the local community to identify priorities. The JSNA covers two core functions of commissioning.

1   To commission the amount of healthcare activity required (e.g. numbers of operations, admissions, attendances at A&E, for outpatients, etc.).
2   To commission the quality of care required, by specifying and monitoring standards (with measures such as infections, rates of venous thromboembolism, or readmissions within 30 days of discharge). NICE's role is to advise the future NHS Commissioning Board on the relevant standards.

Practice-level commissioning gives individual GPs and practice nurses more say in how the NHS provides services to their patients, so that services better reflect patients' preferences.

BOX 8.1 Providers from which services are commissioned

Provider trusts
- Acute trusts
- Mental health trusts
- Ambulance trusts
- Community services trusts

Primary care services
- General practitioners
- Dental practitioners
- Community pharmacists
- Community optometrists

Directly provided services
- Community hospitals
- Community nursing teams

NHS trusts provide healthcare services that have been commissioned by PCTs and practice-based commissioners. Trusts generally concentrate on one work area: acute care, mental health, learning disability, community or ambulance. All trusts have a legal duty to break even, earn a specific financial return on capital and meet minimum quality standards.

FOUNDATION TRUSTS

Since 2004, trusts have been able to apply to change their status to NHS foundation trusts. As of 1 April 2010 there were 129 NHS foundation trusts in the United Kingdom. The Department of Health wants all trusts to become foundation trusts in the next few years. Foundation trusts differ from NHS trusts in being independent from strategic health authority / Department of Health control. They are regulated by Monitor, who reports directly to parliament and have increased financial obligations to maintain surpluses. In return, they have the freedom to keep receipts from capital sales, and decide how to meet national targets rather than being performance-managed. They can borrow money under strict conditions and set their own terms and conditions for staff locally. In other words they operate more like private providers.

NEW PROVIDERS

In the United Kingdom, there have always been healthcare providers other than the NHS. However, historically these providers have mainly provided care to those who either had private insurance or paid directly and there was very little provision of

NHS care. Since 1997 many other providers have entered the NHS market; they can be divided into three groups:

Private sector

This sector is managed and owned by private companies. It was established to provide secondary care to insurance companies, and it increasingly provides NHS services by winning contracts to provide specific services via the commissioning process.

Third sector

This includes voluntary groups and charitable organisations, cooperatives, trusts, community interest groups and foundations, working, for instance, in the mental health and substance misuse sectors. These groups often bridge the gap between care sectors.

Social enterprises

Social enterprises are organisations that are run along business lines, but where any profits are reinvested into the community or into service developments. Encouraging social enterprise in health- and social care is a central part of recent and planned NHS reforms.

ARM'S-LENGTH BODIES

There are many arm's-length bodies that play important roles within the NHS. They are frequently the subject of review, to ensure that they continue to be required and are 'fit for purpose'. Some examples are identified here.

Regulating the health service

The NHS has a number of different regulators for different purposes. The main ones are listed below.

Care Quality Commission

The Care Quality Commission replaced the Healthcare Commission, Mental Health Act Commission and the Commission for Social Care Inspection in April 2009. Its role is to regulate the quality of both healthcare and adult social care in England (visit www.cqc.org.uk).

Monitor

This body assesses trusts applying for foundation trust status to ensure they are legally constituted, financially sound and well governed. The regulator ensures that, once authorised, NHS foundation trusts continue to meet the terms of their licence. Monitor reports directly to parliament (visit www.monitor-nhsft.gov.uk).

Medicines and Healthcare products Regulatory Agency

This agency monitors the safety of new medications and products and licenses new medicinal products (visit www.mhra.gov.uk).

Regulation of professionals

Individual professionals within the NHS are also regulated, through professional regulatory bodies, such as the General Medical Council, the Nursing and Midwifery Council, the Health Professions Council, the General Dental Council, the General Optical Council and the General Osteopathic Council.

Standard-setting bodies

The National Institute for Health and Clinical Excellence (NICE) is the main standard-setting body for the NHS. It has several key roles.

➤ To advise on the cost-effectiveness of treatments and technologies, including drugs and interventional procedures, and recommend whether they should be provided for NHS patients.

➤ To develop guidelines on the most effective evidence-based treatment for diseases and conditions.

➤ To provide advice on evidence-based practice for improving the health of communities through public health and other interventions.

➤ To make up-to-date evidence readily available to all healthcare practitioners (mainly through the 'NHS Evidence' website).

➤ To advise DH (and the NHS Commissioning Board) on quality standards for NHS commissioning.

Service delivery organisations

These include the Health Protection Agency (HPA), which delivers services to protect communities against infectious disease and environmental hazards, and includes locally responsive health protection advice and interventions, support to NHS organisations (such as trusts in healthcare-associated infection or Legionnaires' disease outbreaks), national surveillance and epidemiological investigation of new and existing infections and specialist functions such as radiological protection. The HPA will become part of the new national public health service.

THE INTERMEDIATE TIER

Strategic health authorities (SHAs) currently form the intermediate tier in the NHS, coordinating and managing the performance of the NHS locally. They occupy the middle tier between the Department of Health and local trusts and PCTs. There are 10 SHAs in England, which are currently responsible for:

➤ leading the NHS, including developing strategic plans for improving health services in their region

➤ ensuring local health services are accessible, of a high quality and performing well

➤ increasing the capacity and capability of local health services so they can provide more and higher-quality services

➤ ensuring national priorities and policies – for example, programmes for

improving cancer services – are explained and integrated into local health
service plans

➤ facilitating local NHS organisations to work together where pooling of regional
resources is required

➤ developing the NHS workforce, and overseeing professional training and
development

➤ holding commissioners of NHS care to account for performance.

They are due to be abolished in 2013 as part of the Coalition's drive to reduce bureaucracy but many of their functions will need to be provided from a similar tier.

LOCAL AUTHORITIES

Care for many people with long-term needs, particularly older people, needs to be
well coordinated with social care, since people with these needs require social support to live independently in the community; otherwise they require more NHS
care. Social care provision is via county and unitary local authorities, and NHS and
social care are interdependent. Better social care reduces demand on NHS services
and vice versa. The same is the case for children's services (in local authorities these
include social care for children and education under a director of children's services).

A variety of partnership arrangements (usually termed 'local strategic partnerships') underpin collaboration between the NHS and local authorities. The Coalition
government plans to develop 'health and well-being boards' in each county and unitary authority, which will have responsibility for joint strategic needs assessments,
approval of GP commissioning plans and coordination of approaches to improve
health across communities among directors of public health, directors of social care
and directors of children's services. GP commissioners will have a statutory duty of
partnership to these boards, which will be able to refer GP commissioning group
plans to the Secretary of State if they are not satisfied with them.

PUBLIC HEALTH

The public health system has been through many changes over recent years, but is
a critical part of improving health in communities. Evidence suggests that about
half of the improvement in health (measured by increased life expectancy) is due to
healthcare, and half due to factors outside of the NHS (wider determinants such as
lifestyle, education, employment and housing).[3]

Public health has three core elements: improving health (using evidence-based
interventions in communities to improve the wider determinants of health), health
protection (protecting communities from infectious disease and environmental hazards) and acting to improve health (and other) service – for example, by advising
commissioners on local health needs and effective interventions.

Currently, health protection is the principal responsibility of the Health Protection
Agency, which supports local NHS organisations, directors of public health (DPHs)

and local government. Health improvement and service public health are delivered locally through DPHs in PCTs, most jointly appointed to local authorities, supported by national programmes such as that on tobacco control. The Coalition government is moving the local DPH role wholly into local government, acting as the 'fount of all wisdom' on the health of the local community and able to influence NHS and social care services, children's services, environment, education, economy and health through the health and well-being board. A new national public health service is being created, taking on the functions of the Health Protection Agency, some functions of the Food Standards Agency and the National Treatment Agency for substance misuse. Public Health England will run national programmes for health improvement, develop evidence, support DPHs in their local authority roles and provide public health support for the NHS Commissioning Board.[4]

COMPLAINTS AND LITIGATION

All organisations learn from complaints and in recent years the number of complaints against staff within the NHS have been rising. How are they handled? The Patient Advice Liaison Service (PALS) can help with their resolution, or refer to the complaints manager (all NHS bodies must have one). First steps should be informal – talking directly with the people involved with a written record. The NHS Constitution states that people should receive a timely and appropriate response. The Independent Complaints and Advocacy Service (ICAS) provides free advice and assistance for making complaints. Other options include independent professional advice, independent review and mediation. The Parliamentary and Health Service Ombudsman may become involved if local processes have been exhausted.

BOX 8.2 Top 10 NHS complaints

- Safety/effectiveness of clinical practice
- Poor communication/lack of information
- Poor response to a complaint
- Patient's experience of care
- Clinical treatment
- Delay or cancellation of appointment
- Attitude of staff
- Lack of access to personal records
- Access to services and waiting times
- Lack of carer/relative involvement

The NHS Litigation Authority (NHSLA) is responsible for handling negligence claims (including employee negligence) made against member NHS bodies in England.

NHS finance

The budget for the NHS in 2008/09 was £96 billion and will rise to about £110 billion in 2010/11. Most money comes from general taxation and National Insurance (NHS portion) receipts (*see* Figure 8.3). A small proportion comes from other sources, such as:

➤ treatment charges (including prescriptions)
➤ dental charges
➤ charges for road traffic and personal injury victims (money claimed from insurers)
➤ overseas visitors
➤ capital receipts.

Spending limits for government departments are the outcome of periodic comprehensive spending reviews (CSR) announced by Treasury. For the 4 years to 2014, spending on the NHS is to be cut from an annual increase of 6% to 0.4%. As part of the CSR the DH enters into a set of agreements with Treasury regarding what they will deliver for the money; these agreements are called public service agreements (PSAs). They set out specific targets and aims towards which the DH will work.

In conclusion, it is not clear whether the Coalition government's policies will achieve their objectives. Proponents of healthcare markets point to evidence of improvements in efficiency at the time of the introduction of the quasi-market in the 1990s.[5] However, there is a clear danger that 'supplier-induced demand' will

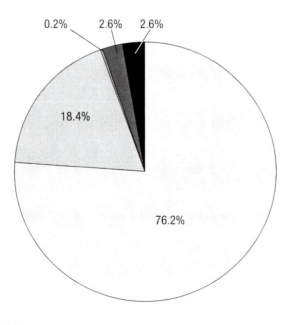

FIGURE 8.3 NHS finance sources pie chart: general taxation 76.2%, National Insurance 18.4%, capital receipts 0.2%, charges 2.6%, interest and loan repayments 2.6%

result from the introduction of fee-for-service incentives leading to an oversupply of expensive hospital care. Furthermore, hospitals may prioritise those services from which they make a financial surplus, rather than those that might most benefit their population's health. The commissioning function within primary care organisations will need to be strengthened to prevent hospitals increasing their activity at the expense of community-based models of care.

REFERENCES

1 McCay L, Jonas S. *A Junior Doctor's Guide to the NHS*. London: NHS Medical Directorate, Department of Health; 2009.
2 Secretary of State for Health. *Equity and Excellence: liberating the NHS*. London: Department of Health; 2010.
3 Wanless D. *Securing our Future: taking a long-term view*. Final report. London: HM Treasury; 2002.
4 Department of Health. *Healthy Lives, Healthy People: our strategy for public health in England*. The Stationery Office; 2010.
4 Le Grand J, Mays N, Mulligan J. *Learning from the NHS Internal Market: a review of the evidence*. London: The King's Fund; 1998.

CHAPTER 9

Change management in the NHS

Q: How do you effect change to health services?

This chapter asks you to think of the myriad influences – internal and external to the health service – that are affecting your job. Surveying the NHS as a whole, two features are immediately apparent. The first is its extraordinary complexity as ever more sophisticated technology is developed to meet an ever-expanding range of health problems. A second feature of modern healthcare is how fast new technologies and services are evolving. Leaders and managers in the NHS are therefore mostly concerned with the management of change.

A simple model of how any health service works is shown in Figure 9.1 and these drivers are examined in turn below. First, we consider the many changing demands faced by the NHS. We have noted already how a succession of reforms are changing health professionals' roles. This, in turn, is affecting how care is provided both in hospitals and in the community. We go on to look at how change is planned and promoted.

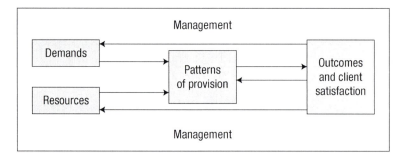

FIGURE 9.1 A simple model of the key components of a healthcare system

CHANGING NEEDS AND DEMANDS

Many studies have demonstrated that health services deal with only a small proportion of the health problems present in a given population. The term 'system iceberg' was coined to draw attention to this fact.[1] Health problems are passed through a series of filters starting with the individual judging whether the problem should be presented to health services. A second filter is the primary care professional – usually the GP – who will manage over 90% of problems presented to primary care. Hospital consultants, in turn, will decide on further investigation, treatment or admission. Of course, the holes in the filters at each of these levels vary, reflecting individuals' varying tolerance of uncertainty. Some patients come more readily to doctors than others; GPs vary in their referral practice, just as hospital doctors' practice varies also.

The central point, as we have seen earlier, is that the pattern of healthcare provided largely reflects the decisions made by relatively autonomous health professionals rather than the policy of governments or managers. That said, three particular forces place pressure on all health systems.

1 *Demographic change* – by 2020, one in four of the population will be aged 65 years and older, rising from one in six today. On average, people in this age group consume five times the national average of health resources. People aged 85 or over are 14 times more likely to be admitted to hospital for medical reasons than young adults aged 16 to 39 years. At an individual level, care at the end of life constitutes about three-quarters of all healthcare used over a lifespan.[2]

2 *Technological innovation* – within 10 years, there are likely to be advances in nanotechnology, robotics and genetic screening and manipulation; within 20 years, in biotechnology drugs, electromedical implants and stem cell technology. The rate of learning about the biological basis of health and disease is providing opportunities undreamed of just a decade ago. Pharmaceutical companies are only the most prominent producers of endlessly evolving medical advances.

However, the real value of much new technology for diagnosis or treatment is debatable. Technology is often not properly evaluated before its introduction and may not be cost-effective or efficient. The National Institute for Health and Clinical Excellence (NICE) was established to undertake appraisal of new health technologies and address this problem. High-tech specialities supported by consumer and commercial interest groups such as drug companies can distort our service spending at the expense of so-called 'Cinderella specialities', such as psychiatry or geriatrics, which may be less technology-dependent but are, nevertheless, labour-intensive.

The cost of technical innovations in healthcare will continue to increase; the government accepts that an annual increase of 1% in real expenditure across the NHS is necessary to keep pace with such changes.

3 *Consumer demand* – in theory, it may be possible to assuage the public's demand for healthcare interventions. For example, there may be a finite limit to any population's requirements for hip replacement surgery. In practice, as governments find to their detriment, there is no limit to what the public may perceive to be 'necessary' healthcare.

Beyond more choice, however, people are now increasingly seeking control of their services. This is seen most clearly in social care, where the idea of 'self-directed support' and personal budgets are challenging the traditional model of care planning by a care manager. The future is likely to see more involvement of people in the public services they use; greater weight accorded to their views; the end of deference to health professionals and bureaucracy.

No amount of public funding can ever allay the sense that is more is needed. Expenditure on healthcare in the United States is already greater in terms of proportion of gross domestic product (GDP) than for any other country in the world – and it continues to increase. Paradoxically, consumer demands seem to be greater where more is already spent. In developing countries, where expectations are lower and other more basic needs go unmet, the demand for healthcare may be less pressing.

The NHS faces a long period of austerity. This follows a decade of unprecedented growth during which health spending expressed as a proportion of GDP has risen to almost 10%, close to the European average. What will this mean for the service? There is likely to be a period of major reductions in capital investment in the fabric of the service from public funds, further attempts to stimulate private sector investment, combined with pay constraint, rationalisation of 'back-office' functions and growing plurality of care provision.

Nevertheless, UK politicians are keenly aware of the priority the electorate attaches to spending on the NHS. While public support has fluctuated in recent years, the NHS retains its symbolic place at the centre of the welfare state. Surveys reaffirm the public's commitment to a tax-funded healthcare system. They also confirm that access to healthcare or waiting times (whether to see a GP, for outpatient appointments or operations) is the public's first priority. As we shall see, this may create conflicts of strategic interest when access targets are used as a measure of quality of care.

PLANNING CHANGE

Introducing a new service or changing an existing service in response to the kind of drivers we have discussed is difficult. Most people will initially resist change even if the results are likely to benefit them. The process of change is about helping people within an organisation or a system change the way they work and interact with others in the system. The ability to plan and manage change is an essential leadership skill.

In Section I we talked about strategy. This is at the heart of the change process: assessing needs, setting priorities and defining the actions to address them. Questions to ask when developing a strategy are listed in Table 9.1.

THE PSYCHOLOGY OF CHANGE

Fundamental to change is the management of people, and an understanding of how they will react is invaluable. Everett Rogers' classic model (*see* Figure 9.2) of how

TABLE 9.1 What should a strategy for a new service address?

How do we make the case?	• Assess local needs taking account of national strategies.
What are we aiming to do?	• Clarify aims, objectives and desired outcomes.
	• Define local standards and set targets.
How do we engage with partners including patients and public?	• Involve all those who are affected by the strategy including clinicians, managers and other staff in the NHS and in partner organisations.
	• Identify who will support and who will oppose it; develop an approach to overcoming this opposition.
How can we make change happen?	• Securing change is the core of the work and needs to be addressed in the planning stage.
	• Include a description of the actions that are required, and an assessment of the resource implications of putting the new service into place with clear financial plans.
How do we know we have done what we wanted to do?	• Evaluate impact by demonstrating achievement against the standards and targets through monitoring routine data and special studies.
How do we make successful change become normal practice?	• The change in practice needs to be sustained to ensure that it becomes routine, as people tend to revert to their old ways of working.
	• This requires individuals to change the way they do things – continuing education, appropriate management strategies, alterations to the work environment, with a process of ongoing monitoring/audit/feedback, may all be required.

people take up innovation helps to explain different people's responses to change.[3] This was based on observations on how farmers took up hybrid seed corn in Iowa. The model describes the differential rate of uptake of an innovation, in order to target promotion of the product, and labels people according to their place on the uptake curve. Rogers' original model described the 'late adopters' as 'laggards' but this seems a pejorative term when there may be good reasons not to take up the innovation. How soon after their introduction, for example, should nurses and doctors be prescribing new, usually more expensive, inhalers for asthma?

Individuals' 'change type' may depend on the particular change they are adopting. This depends on the perceived benefits, the perceived obstacles and the motivation to make the change. People are more likely to adopt an innovation:

➤ that provides a *relative advantage* compared with old ideas
➤ that is *compatible* with the existing value system of the adopter
➤ that is readily understood by the adopters (*less complexity*)
➤ that may be experienced on a limited basis (*more trialability*)
➤ where the results of the innovation are more easily noticed by other potential adopters (*observability*).

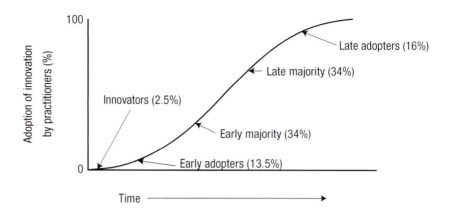

FIGURE 9.2 Diffusion of innovation

Pharmaceutical companies use this model in their approaches to general practition-ers. The local sales representatives know from the information they have about GPs in their area whether a GP is an early adopter. Early adopters are often opinion lead-ers in a community. Early on in the process of promotion they will target those GPs with personal visits, whereas they may send the late adopters an information leaflet only, as those GPs will not consider change until more than 80% of their colleagues have taken up the new product.

Anyone hoping to change people's behaviour is looking for the 'tipping point'.[4] This is the point or threshold at which an idea or behaviour takes off, moving from uncommon to common. You see it in many areas of life: new technologies like the uptake of mobile phones, fashion garments, books or TV programmes. The phar-maceutical industry looks for that point for GPs' prescribing of their drug, or for customers choosing their product when buying over the counter. The change in behaviour is contagious, like infectious disease epidemics; a social epidemic. Using the model of diffusion, the tipping point comes at the point between the early adop-ters and the early majority. It applies also to changing the behaviour of professionals and the public.

This same technique can be used with staff going through a process of change. It is important to identify change types and opinion leaders. Knowing likely opponents is important because if they can be persuaded to support the change they are likely to become important advocates. Understanding people's psychological reaction to change is a key to helping overcome their resistance.

TOOLS FOR HELPING HEALTH PROFESSIONALS CHANGE

Changes to systems, structures and culture are underpinned by changes in the way people within the organisation behave. There is a body of knowledge about what helps professional staff change the way they work. There are many approaches to securing change in the behaviour of healthcare professionals, including:

➤ guidelines dissemination
➤ local opinion leaders
➤ clinical audit and feedback
➤ educational outreach
➤ continuing professional development
➤ patient-mediated approaches
➤ patient-specific reminders – for example, computer prompts
➤ financial levers/contracting.

Numerous systematic reviews have examined what works in practice and organisational change.[5] These are summarised in Box 9.1 but can also be summed up in one aphorism: there is no 'magic bullet'. Most interventions are effective under some circumstances; none is effective under all circumstances. A diagnostic analysis of the individual and the context must be performed before selecting a method for altering individual practitioner behaviour. Interventions based on the assessment of potential barriers are more likely to be effective.

BOX 9.1 Evidence of effectiveness of interventions to change professional behaviour

There is good evidence to support the following.
- *Multifaceted interventions* – by targeting different barriers to change, these are more likely to be effective than single interventions.
- *Educational outreach* – this is generally effective in changing prescribing behaviour in US settings. Ongoing trials will provide rigorous evidence about the effectiveness of this approach in UK settings.
- *Reminder systems* – these are generally effective for a range of behaviours.

There are mixed effects in the following.
- *Audit and feedback* – these need to be used selectively.
- *Opinion leaders* – these need to be used selectively.

There is little evidence to support the following.
- *Passive dissemination of guidelines* – though there is some evidence to support use of guidelines if tailored to local needs and associated with reminders.

We considered various theoretical approaches to managing change in Section I, Chapter 5. The scenarios in Chapter 12 take you through practical examples from the NHS.

REFERENCES

1 Last JM. The iceberg: completing the clinical picture in general practice. *Lancet*. 1963; **2**: 28–31.

2 National Audit Office. *End of Life Care*. London: NAO, The Stationery Office; 2008.

3 Rogers E. *The Diffusion of Innovation*. 4th ed. New York: Free Press; 1995.

4 Gladwell M. *The Tipping Point: how little things can make a big difference*. London: Abacus; 2000.

5 Cochrane Library review topic: Effective Practice and Organisation of Care. Available at: www.cochrane.org/reviews/en/topics/61.html (accessed 21 January 2011).

CHAPTER 10

Improving quality of healthcare

Q: How would you measure the quality of the care you provide?

How do we know whether our interventions are having the desired effect? Clinicians can monitor the impact of treatments on an individual patient basis but how do we examine the impact of a new service or screening programme? In this chapter, we will look first at what is meant by quality of care and how it is measured. We then consider how quality of care is promoted across the National Health Service (NHS) as a whole.

WHAT IS QUALITY?

Quality in healthcare means doing the right thing, at the right time, in the right way, to the right person – and having the best possible result. A more formal framework is provided by Maxwell, who described six dimensions to quality:[1]

1 effectiveness (achieves intended benefit)
2 acceptability (satisfies reasonable expectations)
3 efficiency (resources not oversupplied to some patients to the detriment of others)
4 accessibility (those who need services will receive them)
5 equity (resources are fairly shared)
6 relevance (treatments are appropriate to their particular target groups).

Of course, it is not only health professionals who are interested in the quality of care they provide – as media interest in medical mishaps reminds us. Managers in hospitals and health authorities are charged to monitor quality as part of clinical governance (see p. 81). Whether as users or voters, the general population have great interest in the quality of healthcare and may have different priorities from doctors. For example, they may place clear information, caring communication and outcomes that improve activities of daily living higher up their list than technical aspects of care, which may be difficult for them to assess.

Quality has been defined as 'the degree to which health services for individuals and populations increase the likelihood of desired health outcomes and are consistent with current professional knowledge'.[2] 'Desired health outcomes' is a key phrase as it deliberately does not specify who is doing the desiring. It implicitly accepts that different people will want different outcomes.

BOX 10.1 Scenario

A 72-year-old woman with osteoarthritis of her left hip is booked for a total hip operation. She also suffers from diabetes and high blood pressure.
- List as many aspects of good-quality care in this situation as you can.
- Who should be involved in assessing the quality of her care?
- Describe the likely concerns of the different individuals and groups involved.

Desired health outcomes may be different for managers, patients and clinicians. Managers are rightly concerned with efficiency, and seek to maximise the population health gain through best use of an inevitably limited budget. Clinicians are more focused on effectiveness, and want the treatment that works best for each of their patients. Patients clearly want treatment that works, and also place a high priority on how the treatment is delivered. Coulter has described the following healthcare aspirations of patients.[3]

➤ Fast access to reliable health advice.
➤ Effective treatment delivered by trusted professionals.
➤ Participation in decisions and respect for preferences.
➤ Clear, comprehensible information and support for self-care.
➤ Attention to physical and environmental needs.
➤ Emotional support, empathy and respect.
➤ Involvement of, and support for, family and carers.
➤ Continuity of care and smooth transitions.

The range of different desired outcomes above demonstrates the multidimensional nature of quality. The first stage in any attempt to measure quality is to think about what dimensions of quality should be measured.

CAN QUALITY BE MEASURED?

Evaluation has been defined as 'a process that attempts to determine as systematically and objectively as possible the relevance, effectiveness and impact of activities in the light of their objectives, e.g. evaluation of structure, process and outcome, clinical trials, quality of care'.[4] Where do we start when thinking about evaluation of a service in the NHS? Avedis Donabedian distinguished four elements:[5]

1 structure (buildings, staff, equipment)
2 process (all that is done to patients)
3 outputs (immediate results of medical intervention)
4 outcomes (gains in health status).

Thus, for example, early evaluation of the new national screening programme for colonic cancer will need to consider:

➤ the volume and costs of new equipment (colonoscopic, radiographic, histopathological), staff and buildings (structure)

➤ the numbers of patients screened, coverage rates within a defined age range, numbers of true and false positives (process)

➤ number of cancers identified, operations performed (outputs)

➤ complication rates, colonic cancer incidence, prevalence and mortality rates (outcomes).

This distinction is helpful because for many interventions it may be difficult to obtain robust data on health outcomes unless large numbers are scrutinised over long periods. For example, evaluating the quality of hypertension management within a general practice, you may be reliant on intermediate outcome or process measures (the proportion of the appropriate population screened, treated and adequately controlled) as a proxy for the health status outcomes. The assumption here is that evidence from larger-scale studies showing that control of hypertension reduces subsequent death rates from heart disease will be reflected in your own practice population's health experience.

Some dimensions of quality, such as clinical effectiveness, are more straight-forward to define and measure quantitatively than 'softer' dimensions such as patient-centred healthcare. There remain concerns that attempts to measure some-thing as complex as healthcare quality may undermine professionalism and the doctor–patient relationship. A more widely held view is that measurement is an essential component of quality improvement. If we do not measure quality, we can-not know whether health services are achieving the level of population health benefit of which they are potentially capable.

APPROACHES TO QUALITY MEASUREMENT

Health systems internationally are using more quantitative measures of quality, usually the rates of delivery of effective healthcare processes. Delivered healthcare is compared with the healthcare that should have been delivered, sometimes referred to as 'indicated care'. Indicated care can be set out in guidelines such as those published by the National Institute for Health and Clinical Excellence (NICE), the Scottish Intercollegiate Guidelines Network (SIGN) and the US Preventive Services Task Force (USPSTF) in the United States.

A good example of the method by which standards of care are developed is the RAND/UCLA appropriateness method.[6] This was developed in response to the lack of randomised controlled clinical trial data on many interventions, and the prob-lems with interpreting sometimes contradictory trial results for use in routine care. It combines research data with clinical expertise, and involves the following stages.

➤ Identifying clinical area(s) of care for quality assessment.

➤ Conducting a systematic review of care in the relevant clinical area(s).

➤ Drafting quality indicators.
➤ Presenting draft quality indicators and their evidence base to a clinical panel for a modified Delphi process. (The Delphi process typically involves asking panel members to anonymously rate the draft indicators for validity over two rounds, with face-to-face discussion between rounds.)
➤ Approving a final set of indicators.

The quality standards produced by methods such as this can be used to assess the quality of care in a single clinic or a whole health system. An example of quality assessment on a very large scale is the payment of incentives to general practitioners in the United Kingdom on the basis of their performance against quality indicators. Table 10.1 gives examples of indicators from the British general practitioners' contract, the so-called Quality and Outcomes Framework (QOF).[7]

PROBLEMS WITH QUALITY
Problems with healthcare can be grouped into one of three broad categories: (1) underuse, (2) overuse and (3) misuse, all of which are amenable to action.[8] Effective healthcare can be underused, so that people miss out on opportunities to

TABLE 10.1 Domains and indicators from the QOF

Clinical domain	No. of indicators	Example of indicator in each clinical domain
Hypertension	3	The percentage of patients with hypertension in whom there is a record of blood pressure in the previous nine months
Asthma	4	The percentage of patients aged eight and over diagnosed as having asthma from 1 April with measures of variability or reversibility
Depression	3	In those patients with a new diagnosis of depression, recorded between the preceding 1 April to 31 March, the percentage of patients who have had an assessment of severity at the outset of treatment using an assessment tool validated for use in primary care
Chronic kidney disease (CKD)	5	The percentage of patients on the CKD register with hypertension who are treated with an angiotensin converting enzyme inhibitor (ACE-I) or angiotensin receptor blocker (ARB) (unless a contraindication or side effects are recorded)
Smoking indicators	2	The percentage of patients with any or any combination of the following conditions: coronary heart disease, stroke or TIA, hypertension, diabetes, COPD or asthma who smoke whose notes contain a record that smoking cessation advice or referral to a specialist service, where available, has been offered within the previous 15 months

benefit from it. It can be overused, wasting resources by delivering care to those who do not need it, or where the potential for harm exceeds the benefit. Misuse is where patients suffer avoidable complications of surgery or medication. An example of misuse is a patient who suffers a rash after receiving penicillin as treatment for an infection, despite having a known allergy to penicillin.

We know effective healthcare is underused. Many effective interventions are only received by half of the people who should receive them.[9] There is also great variability in the quality of care experienced by different populations, by illness, age, sex, race, wealth, geographic location, insurance coverage. Julian Tudor Hart drew attention to inequalities in care with his famous Inverse Care Law nearly 40 years ago.[10]

> The availability of good medical care tends to vary inversely with the need for it in the population served. This . . . operates more completely where medical care is most exposed to market forces, and less so where such exposure is reduced. The market distribution of medical care is a primitive and historically outdated social form, and any return to it would further exaggerate the maldistribution of medical resources.

We also know that care is overused. Wennberg and colleagues first documented the wide variations in care received by similar populations. They showed that healthcare is often driven by the availability of specialist services, rather than by the health needs of the population, with no detectable difference in health outcomes.[11] This variation in quantity of healthcare with no apparent relationship with quality implies that some healthcare is overused. People are receiving more care than they have the capacity to benefit from.

Harm resulting from misuse of healthcare is a major problem. Adverse drug events have been shown to cause considerable morbidity, mortality and cost in the United Kingdom and the United States.[12] This patient safety problem is the flip side of quality; greater attention is now devoted to reporting, analysing and learning from adverse incidents and 'near misses' involving NHS patients. The following four factors aggravate our attempts to improve the quality of healthcare.

1 The growing complexity of science and technology. Our ability to deliver safe, effective healthcare cannot keep up with rapid advances in science and medical treatments.
2 The increase in chronic conditions. People are now living longer, and chronic conditions are the major cause of disability and death; they consume the majority of healthcare resources in developed countries.
3 Poorly organised delivery systems. Most healthcare systems are still designed to deal primarily with acute health problems and lack an effective chronic care model.
4 Constraints on exploiting the revolution in information technology.[2]

None of these reasons for widespread quality problems lays the blame on individual clinicians making mistakes. They emphasise the important truism that quality is often a property of health systems, and not simply of the health professionals in the system. Human beings will always make occasional errors, and experience from other industries has shown that dramatic quality improvement can occur when systems are designed that do not rely on humans avoiding mistakes.

HOW CAN QUALITY OF CARE BE IMPROVED?

Many different approaches to quality improvement in healthcare have been tried in the past, with varying levels of success. They can be broadly classified into three groups, as summarised in Table 10.2.[13]

Regulation and standards

A robust regulatory framework is important for assuring a basic standard of healthcare, and regulation of medical professionals is a central component of quality improvement in nearly all countries. The three main purposes of professional regulation are to set minimally acceptable standards of care, to provide accountability of professionals to patients and payers and to improve quality of care by providing guidance about best practice.[13]

In the United Kingdom, the General Medical Council regulates doctors, and is currently adapting to a new environment where greater levels of public accountability are required. Standards are developed for the NHS through national service frameworks. The NICE evaluates new technologies and develops guidelines. A popular misconception is that more guidelines and protocols will avoid major harmful incidents. A reliance on ever more detailed frameworks could erode the ability of health workers and their managers to make judgements and act with ingenuity when they encounter problems. The Care Quality Commission assesses the performance of healthcare organisations. The involvement of patients and public is promoted at both a local and a national level. Annual surveys of users form part of the monitoring process. The National Patient Safety Agency was created to coordinate the efforts of all those involved in healthcare and, more important, to learn from patient safety incidents occurring in the NHS (*see* Chapter 8).

Education and audit

The dominant approach for health professionals has been education and audit, with limited success. Education and audit are common requirements for regulation, but

TABLE 10.2 Approaches to quality improvement in healthcare

Type of approach	Example
Regulation and standards	American Board of Medical Specialties in the United States
	General Medical Council in the United Kingdom
Education and audit	Royal Colleges, professional organisations
Market and financial	Payment of British general practitioners according to achievement of performance indicators

go beyond the requirements of regulation in that they seek to go beyond a minimum standard, and strive for excellence. Education has traditionally been professionally led, and is seen by many as an obligation of professional status. Professional organisations, such as the Royal Colleges in the United Kingdom, have been influential in setting high standards and encouraging audit.

The concept of the 'learning organisation' remains influential. Peter Senge suggests that a learning organisation is one in which it is impossible not to learn because learning is so much part of everything the organisation does.[14] He borrowed on earlier models of organisational learning developed by Chris Argyris and Donald Schon.[15] The latter's work has been particularly influential among educationalists for bringing reflection into the centre of what health professionals do.[16] He contrasted the technical rationality underpinning roles such as doctoring from the messy uncertainties of actual practice. Schon distinguished reflection in action (the artistic, intuitive judgements using tacit and instinctive knowledge) from reflection on action afterwards (say, on the norms that underlie a judgement or on the strategies implicit in a pattern of behaviour); both are required to cope with the inchoate and unexpected realities of work day-to-day. Consider how much medical care deals with illnesses that defy conventional categorisations.

CLINICAL AUDIT

The clinical audit cycle refers to the monitoring of performance against predefined standards (*see* Figures 10.1 and 10.2). Measurement of one's performance against defined criteria can be demanding but the real challenge is to make necessary adjustments and re-evaluate your performance – in other words, to complete the cycle.

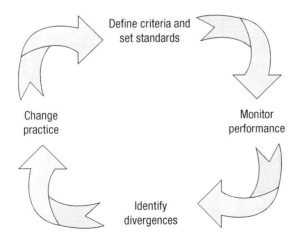

Define criteria and
set standards

Monitor
performance

Identify
divergences

Change
practice

FIGURE 10.1 The clinical audit cycle

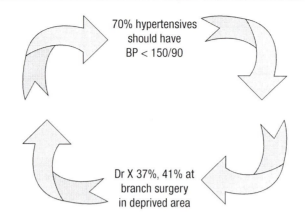

FIGURE 10.2 A routine example of clinical audit from frontline general practice

BOX 10.2 Audit example

One criterion used to assess the quality of care provided for people with hypertension is the proportion of patients whose blood pressure (BP) lies below 150/90 (140/85 for people with diabetes). Under their new contract general practice teams are rewarded for achieving a target of 70% of people with hypertension thus controlled (the standard). In this instance, the practice was surprised to find that they were only achieving 64% coverage. On closer examination of data, it transpired that coverage among hypertensive patients attending the branch surgery sited on a deprived estate was only 41%. Furthermore, only 37% of the patients of Doctor X who works predominantly from this site were adequately controlled.

Various interventions were made to tackle these divergences. The clinical audit lead decided to monitor performance more closely. Patients whose blood pressure remained elevated and who had not been seen in the last 6 months were contacted by letter and asked to attend surgery. Doctor X was provided with a copy of the practice hypertension protocol (based on NICE guidelines) and asked to dedicate more time to this area of his clinical practice. The records of patients in the target group were tagged electronically so as to ease their identification at opportunistic consultation. More nurse time was channelled to supporting the branch surgery.

Regular monthly monitoring and sharing of the results across the team over the next half year revealed gratifying improvements. Six months later coverage rates among Doctor X's patients under the branch surgery were 62% and 66% respectively; across the practice as a whole the 70% target was achieved.

The Institute for Healthcare Improvement's Plan–Do–Study–Act (PDSA) cycle takes audit one stage further, and is widely used in healthcare (*see* Figure 10.3). The PDSA cycle has four stages, designed to help with the development, testing and implementation of quality improvement plans. The stages are, first, to develop a plan and define the objective (plan); second, to carry out the plan and collect data (do), then analyse the data and summarise what was learned (study). The final stage is to plan the next cycle with necessary modifications (act) (www.ihi.org/ihi).

Examples of other quality improvement methods are listed in Box 10.3.[17]

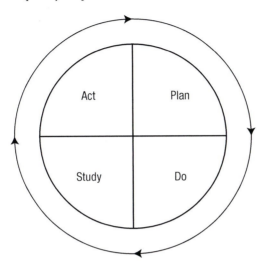

FIGURE 10.3 The Institute for Healthcare Improvement's Plan–Do–Study–Act cycle

BOX 10.3 Examples of quality improvement evaluation methods

Audit and improvement cycles
1   Clinical audit
2   Significant event analysis
3   Plan–Do–Study–Act cycles

Analysis of barriers and facilitators to improvement
1   Discovery (narrative) interviews, focus groups
2   Participant and non-participant observation, naturalistic story gathering (ethnography)
3   Organisational case study
4   Critical to quality (CTQ) trees

Change management
1   WIFM ('what's in it for me') charts
2   Strengths, weaknesses, opportunities, threats (SWOT) or strengths, challenges, opportunities, threats (SCOT) analysis
3   Force field analysis

Transformation methods
1 Process redesign
2 Collective sense making (action research)

Measurement for change
1 Benchmarking
2 Confidence charts or funnel plots

Market and financial

Market-based approaches have been most used in the United States, and rely on an informed consumer exercising choice. An example is the publishing of risk-adjusted mortality rates from coronary artery bypass grafting for hospitals and surgeons in New York State.[18] Importantly, the data were used to inform quality improvement efforts that were associated with statewide reduction in mortality. Following the Bristol inquiry, cardiothoracic surgeons have pioneered similar systems in the United Kingdom. Public release of performance data alone has met with limited success in improving quality – perhaps because the data are not used by the public – unless accompanied by broader improvement programmes.

Payment for performance (P4P) is perhaps the dominant model internationally today. Examples are the Quality and Outcomes Framework (QOF), which provides a quarter of British general practitioners' salaries according to their performance against quality criteria (*see* Table 10.1), and the CQUIN (Commissioning for Quality and Innovation) payment framework, which makes a small percentage of English hospital funding conditional upon quality of care. However, the QOF well illustrates both the gains and less desirable consequences of P4P.[19]

The business world has given us powerful examples of quality improvement initiatives that consider the whole system, and two that have been successfully adopted into healthcare are Six Sigma, invented by Motorola, and Toyota's 'lean manufacturing'. The lean technique entails assessing every process for its value to the patient, to cut waste and inefficiencies and improve patient care.[20] Six Sigma describes the aspiration to reduce error rates to the extremely low level of 3.4 per million.[21] The term Six Sigma comes from a statistical measure of variation, the standard deviation from a normal distribution. The number of 3.4 million comes from the limits for acceptable quality being set to include all observations within six standard deviations of the mean. The statistical terminology can be confusing, but the idea is simple: we should not accept the current common error rates of 50% in healthcare, nor 10% or even 1%, but strive for near-perfect error rates of fewer than 1 in 3.4 million. Proponents of Six Sigma argue that these error rates are achievable in healthcare, just as in manufacturing, and cite anaesthesia as an example of an area that has seen dramatic improvements in safety. Table 10.3 gives examples of the defect rates (which relate to a particular sigma level) in different industries.

The risks of quality improvement should also be considered. Do the benefits outweigh the costs? Disparities in access to healthcare are a problem in all countries, and

TABLE 10.3 Sigma levels and defect rates in different industries

Defects per million	Sigma level	Healthcare examples	Other industry examples
3.4	6		One misspelled word in all books in a small library
5.4		Deaths caused by anaesthesia during surgery	
230	5		Airline fatalities
6210	4		Airline baggage handling Restaurant bills
10 000		1% of all hospitalised patients injured through negligence	
66 800	3		7.6 misspelled words per page in a book
210 000		21% of ambulatory antibiotics for colds	
	2	58% of patients with depression not diagnosed/treated adequately	
790 000	1	79% of heart attack survivors not given beta blockers	

any quality improvement programme may worsen disparities unless the improvement has proportionally greater benefit for the relatively disadvantaged population.

The most important part of any quality improvement initiative is a group of committed people who consistently seek to make healthcare better. Previously, most quality improvement took place in single clinics, in patients with single diseases. However, multilevel approaches to change, that impact on individuals, groups or teams, the organisation as a whole, and the larger environment and system level, have greater chances of success.[22]

CLINICAL GOVERNANCE

A whole-system approach to quality improvement is implicit in the concept of clinical governance described in Chapter 5. A common criticism of much of what doctors do to try to improve the quality of their care is that it is piecemeal and poorly coordinated. *A First Class Service*, published by the Labour government in 1998, contained a blueprint for improving quality, encapsulated in Figure 10.4.

The term 'clinical governance' refers to the framework through which NHS organisations and their staff are accountable for the quality of patient care. It covers the organisations, systems and processes for monitoring and improving services. The different components of clinical governance are listed in Table 10.4.

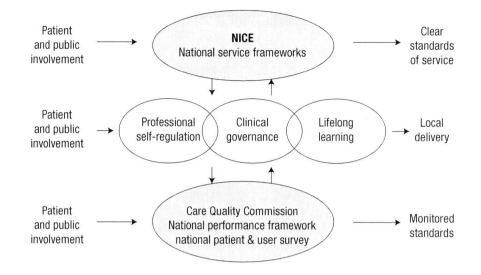

FIGURE 10.4 Standards for the NHS

TABLE 10.4 Elements of clinical governance

Processes for quality improvement	• Patient and public involvement
	• Risk management
	• Clinical audit
	• Clinical effectiveness programmes
	• Staffing and staff management
Staff focus	• Education, training and continuing personal and professional development
Information	• Use of information to support clinical governance and healthcare delivery

EVIDENCE-BASED HEALTHCARE

Few people nowadays question that both policy and practice should be based where possible on high-quality research evidence but evidence-based healthcare is a relatively new phenomenon, really only taking hold in the mid 1990s. Nowadays NICE and other national organisations undertake research on the effectiveness and costs of healthcare interventions to determine health policy in the NHS. The national service frameworks (NSFs) also build on the evidence base to inform clinical practice. These frameworks define the care pathways, activities and outcomes for all elements of a care pathway, from prevention, primary, secondary and tertiary care through to rehabilitation and palliative care. They provide blueprints, therefore, for how care in NSF areas should be delivered in primary care. The statements in the NSFs are graded in terms of the strength of the evidence to support them.

The skills of asking the right question and finding and appraising the evidence should therefore be central for managers as well as for clinicians.[23] Critical appraisal of research literature helps readers:

➤ decide how trustworthy a piece of research is (*validity*)
➤ determine what it is telling us (*results*)
➤ weigh up how useful and important the research will be to the clinician (or manager) and to the patient (*relevance*).

The Critical Appraisal Skills Programme website has critical appraisal checklists for a range of different types of research studies (go to www.phru.nhs.uk/casp/casp.htm).

Evidence has to be derived not only from research on what works but also from research on cost-effectiveness. The NHS does not formally use a threshold cost–benefit ratio to determine whether to invest in a drug or in other interventions. However, in practice, NICE guidance recommends that the NHS should invest in services where the cost per QALY (quality-adjusted life year) is £20 000 to £30 000 or less (*see* Chapter 11).

As well as evidence, there are other factors that need to be taken into account in introducing treatments – for instance, how easily new practice can be implemented, and its acceptability to patients. The decision to provide a treatment is based only partly on evidence. Experience and common sense also have a role in any decisions as do political concerns including the public's views. Take, for example, screening for prostate-specific antigen (PSA). The PSA blood test has been developed as a screening test for prostate cancer. There is insufficient evidence of its effectiveness to introduce the test routinely. However, the government has made the PSA test available on request because of strong public demand for it. Sound judgement is the key to interpreting the evidence and making a decision about how to apply it to your local situation.

It has been possible here only to touch on the burgeoning sciences of quality improvement in healthcare but this exciting area will provide a major focus for medical managers in the coming years.

SUSTAINABLE HEALTHCARE

Finally, efficient use of resources minimises waste and maximises the quantity of high-quality healthcare. Risks to quality, due to misuse of resources, arise both externally and internally. External risk results from using resources in a way that destabilises the foundations of the interconnected economic, societal or environmental world in which the health system operates. Internal risk results from using resources in a way that outstrips supply and threatens economic viability. The NHS is Europe's largest public sector carbon emitter. The NHS has a carbon footprint of 18 million tonnes of CO_2 per year. This is composed of energy (22%), travel (18%) and procurement (60%). Despite an increase in efficiency, the NHS has increased its carbon footprint by 40% since 1990.[24] Doctors have an ethical imperative to help reduce 'in-house' emissions. While healthcare activity (equipment, lighting, heating, cooling, construction, transport and delivery, and so on) is largely powered by fossil fuels, 'internal' system inefficiencies can be highlighted by measuring the carbon waste or footprint of healthcare pathways.[25]

One in eight cars on the road are said to be on NHS-related business. The NHS Sustainable Development Unit aims not only to reduce waste in existing care pathways but also to transform how healthcare is provided. Examples of this are prioritisation of disease prevention, improved integration of primary and secondary care with rewards for outcomes over activity, smart procurement and better use of information and communication technology. Sustainable practice will save money but the health system improvements and co-benefits to patients (health gains from exercise rather than car travel, better diets, etc.) are easily overlooked. Transforming the way we practise will require engaging NHS staff at all levels in a huge change management exercise (*see* Chapter 9).

In conclusion, it is easy to overlook dramatic advances over the last 20 years in our ability to measure quality in healthcare. Bodies such as NICE have brought clarity to quality by distilling the range of guidance available into key markers of high-quality care in different clinical areas. Nowadays, doctors are more likely to report that there is too much rather than too little guidance on what constitutes good practice. High-performing teams are defined by their willingness to measure their own performance and use this information to continually improve. Strong clinical and academic leadership at all levels of the NHS is central to this continual improvement.

REFERENCES

1 Maxwell R. Quality assessment in health. *BMJ*. 1984; **288**: 1470–2.

2 Institute of Medicine (IOM)'s Committee on Health Care in America. *Crossing the Quality Chasm: a new health system for the 21st century.* Washington, DC: National Academy Press; 2001.

3 Coulter A. *Engaging Patients in their Healthcare: how is the UK doing relative to other countries?* Oxford: Picker Institute Europe; 2006.

4 Last JM. *A Dictionary of Epidemiology.* 4th ed. Oxford: Oxford University Press; 2001.

5 Donabedian A. *The Definition of Quality and Approaches to its Assessment.* Ann Arbor, MI: Health Administration Press; 1980.

6 Brook RH, Chassin MR, Fink A, *et al.* A method for the detailed assessment of the appropriateness of medical technologies. *Int J Technol Assess Health Care.* 1986; **2**: 53–63.

7 General Practitioners Committee BMA, The NHS Confederation. *Investing in General Practice: the new general medical services contract.* London: The NHS Confederation; 2003.

8 Chassin M, Galvin RW, the National Roundtable on Healthcare Quality. The urgent need to improve health care quality. *JAMA.* 1998; **280**: 1000–5.

9 McGlynn EA, Asch SM, Adams J, *et al.* The quality of health care delivered to adults in the United States. *N Engl J Med.* 2003; **348**(26): 2635–45.

10 Tudor Hart J. The inverse care law. *Lancet.* 1971; 297: 404–12.

11 Fisher ES, Wennberg D, Stukel T, *et al.* The implications of regional variations in Medicare

spending. Part 1: the content, quality, and accessibility of care. *Ann Intern Med.* 2003; **138**(4): 273–87.

12 Institute of Medicine (IOM)'s Committee on Health Care in America. *To Err Is Human: building a safer health system.* Washington, DC: National Academy Press; 2000.

13 Sutherland K, Leatherman S. Does certification improve medical standards? *BMJ.* 2006; **333**(7565): 439–41.

14 Senge P. *The Fifth Discipline: the art and practice of the learning organisation.* London: Random House Books; 2006.

15 Argyris C, Schon D. *Organisational Learning: a theory of action perspective.* Reading, MA: Addison Wesley; 1978.

16 Schon D. *The Reflective Practitioner: how professionals think in action.* London: Temple Smith; 1973.

17 Siriwardena N. Quality improvement methods for evaluating health care. *Qual Prim Care.* 2009; **17**: 155–9.

18 Chassin MR. Achieving and sustaining improved quality: lessons from New York State and cardiac surgery. *Health Aff (Millwood).* 2002; **21**(4): 40–51.

19 Gillam S, Siriwardena N. *The Quality and Outcomes Framework: transforming general practice.* Radcliffe Publishing: Oxford; 2010.

20 Jones D, Mitchell A. *Lean Thinking for the NHS.* London: NHS Confederation; 2006.

21 Chassin MR. Is health care ready for six sigma quality? *Milbank Q.* 1998; **76**(4): 565–91.

22 Ferlie EB, Shortell SM. Improving the quality of healthcare in the United Kingdom and the United States: a framework for change. *Milbank Q.* 2001; **79**(2): 281–315.

23 Muir Gray JA. *Evidence-based Health Care: how to make health policy and management decisions.* 2nd ed. London: Churchill Livingstone; 2001.

24 Sustainable Development Unit. *Saving Carbon, Improving Health: NHS Carbon Reduction Strategy for England.* London: Department of Health; 2009.

25 Thomas J, Cosford P. Place sustainability at the heart of the quality agenda. *Qual Saf Health Care.* 2010; **19**: 260–1.

CHAPTER 11

Setting priorities in healthcare

Q: How would you allocate limited resources for health services?

National Health Service (NHS) funding has been a source of debate since 1948. William Beveridge, whose epochal report established the NHS, seems to have believed that, once the backlog of health needs were met, funding requirements for the new health service would actually decline. In retrospect, this seems extraordinarily naïve. From very early on, it became clear that the needs of a growing population were putting strains on the NHS. Since then periodic crises of underfunding have characterised this part of the public sector. As we have seen, the most radical 'solution' was the establishment of a market for healthcare in the early 1990s.

In all countries healthcare budgets are finite. In publicly funded health systems, those responsible for procuring healthcare need to be able to explain how taxpayers' money has been spent. Leaders and managers have to make difficult decisions about how to allocate limited resources. Indeed, even if the budget were continuously elastic, people's health needs and demands could still continue to use up the resources available. The ageing population, the growth in costly new treatments and technologies and an increasingly well-informed public mean that the need to prioritise will intensify. The gap between what is demanded and what can be supplied from the public purse leads to the inevitability of rationing.

Decisions are made at both an individual patient and a population level. At an individual level the decision might be should this patient get a prescription for a statin to lower her blood cholesterol and, if so, which statin should it be? At a population level the decision might be will a GP commissioning group employ a heart failure specialist nurse or run an additional sexual health clinic? (*See* Box 11.1.) In the United Kingdom funding decisions are made at various levels. Individual clinicians, managers within primary care organisations and hospitals, managers in strategic health authorities and civil servants in the Department of Health all make decisions that affect what public health and treatment services are available to populations.[1]

How these kinds of decisions are made is the focus of this chapter. We will look briefly at a framework for priority setting and consider what factors should be taken into account when comparing options. This will include an examination of basic health economic concepts.

BOX 11.1 Example of competing demands for limited funding

At the year end there was an additional £100 000 available for commissioning. The hospital identified three competing areas for the resource available.

1 *The waiting list for cataract operations* – one cataract operation costs £715. Investment here would mean that 140 operations could be done, which would improve the vision of that number of older people, enabling them to live independently in the community.

2 *Adults waiting for cochlear implant operations* – investment here would mean that four hard-of-hearing or deaf adults could be helped to hear at a cost of £25 000 per implant with maintenance.

3 *Dementia* – sixty patients with dementia could attend the memory clinic and be given the drug donepezil. Thirty per cent of those taking the drug are thought to benefit, with variable improvements in their quality of life.

Which would you choose – how and why?

A FRAMEWORK FOR SETTING PRIORITIES

Proper consideration of different service options should be systematic. If the answer to any of the following questions is negative, the proposal is unlikely to be a priority for funding.

Is there a need for the service?

Health economists define need as the capacity to benefit so the use of needs assessment is crucial to determining which interventions for which health and healthcare issues are likely to benefit the population most and so become priorities. Populations vary according to age, sex, ethnicity and many other determinants of health. Their needs for health services will vary accordingly.

Is there an effective intervention/service?

If an intervention doesn't work it shouldn't be provided by a publicly funded healthcare organisation. The Cochrane Library can be searched for systematic reviews and other repositories of evidence inform a decision. However, there are many areas of study where the quality and quantity of evidence is limited.

Is the intervention acceptable to users?

Services that are not acceptable to patients or the public may be used inefficiently. When introducing new services, the views of patients and the public should be considered.

Is the service a political priority?

Governments come to power with their own electoral commitments; these will be shaped within the Department of Health. Local electorates may have identified concerns also.

Is the intervention cost-effective?

In a system where healthcare resources are limited, costs must be factored into decision-making. However, money is not the only cost and saving lives is not the only benefit. Costs and benefits should be measured accurately and used to compare different interventions and outcomes.

ECONOMIC EVALUATION

Economic evaluation can be defined as 'the comparative analysis of alternative courses of action in terms of both their costs and consequences'.[2] Costs are generally divided into direct and indirect costs. Direct costs are those associated with the activity (for example, the costs of staff time, drugs and dressings). Indirect costs are more difficult to measure and might include items such as overheads (e.g. heating and lighting) for the building in which the health professionals works. Opportunity costs should be taken into account. The opportunity cost is the amount lost by not using the resource (labour, capital) in its best alternative use. For example, the financial cost of admitting an older patient with influenza and respiratory problems to a surgical ward (due to lack of beds) is relatively low (cost of bed, nursing, etc.). However, the opportunity cost of the admission may be much higher (e.g. cancelled operations, increased waiting lists). Options are rarely simple and the concept of marginal costs is helpful. Increasingly, healthcare interventions make small, additional gains to health. Decisions are generally not whether to have a service or not but whether to improve the existing service in certain ways.

Table 11.1 illustrates the different types of economic evaluation. Cost-minimisation analyses do not count what we gain but assume the benefits of each option are the

TABLE 11.1 Types of evaluation

	Costs measured in	Benefits measured in	Smoking cessation as an example
Cost-minimisation	Money	Not measured	Cost of one clinic compared with cost of two
Cost-effectiveness	Money	Natural units – units relevant to the intervention	Costs per additional quitter
Cost-utility	Money	Comparable units – usually QALYs	Cost per additional QALY* gained for the quitters
Cost–benefit	Money	Money	Here you would need to value the benefits in financial terms

same. This type of analysis is often used in medicines management when alternative drugs having the same clinical indication and effect are compared according to price and the cheapest prescribed. However, it is rarely the case that all consequences are equal. Within a cost-effectiveness analysis we measure the two sets of costs and compare the outcomes in units of relevance for the intervention. This is often lives saved or life years gained. Cost-utility analyses are useful as they measure all outcomes in terms of an index of benefit that is comparable across different types of service. The quality-adjusted life year (QALY) is the most commonly used index of benefit. This allocates a quality of life value (between 1 (perfect health) and 0 (death)) and combines quantity and quality of life to derive the QALY. Although cost-utility analysis allows different types of intervention to be compared, a number of methodological problems remain (*see* Box 11.2) and QALYs are controversial. They can be seen as 'ageist': reduced life expectancy results in lower QALY values so that interventions for older patients may compare poorly with those for young patients. QALYs may disadvantage those already disabled as their quality of life is already lower; interventions for the disabled may yield fewer QALYs than those for healthier people.

BOX 11.2 How a QALY is constructed

A quality-adjusted life year (QALY) combines the quantity and quality of life.[3] It takes 1 year of perfect health-life expectancy to be worth 1 and regards 1 year of less-than-perfect life expectancy as < 1. Patients, the public and professionals are asked to judge the quality value (utility) for 1 year lived with the relevant condition and these values are then used multiplicatively with the number of years lived in this state to give the QALY. For example, an intervention that results in a patient living for an additional 4 years rather than dying within 1 year, but where quality of life for treated and untreated fell from 1 to 0.6 will generate:

- 4 years' extra life @ 0.6 QoL values = 2.4
- less 1 year @ reduced quality = 0.6
- QALYs generated by the intervention = 1.8.

QALYs can, therefore, provide an indication of the benefits gained from a variety of medical procedures in terms of quality of life and additional years for the patient.

Lastly, cost–benefit analyses allow us to choose between diverse uses of public money – for example, on healthcare or education. However, allocating monetary values to all consequences is difficult (how much money is a life saved worth?) and requires complicated methodologies, which are open to challenge.

Thus, types of economic evaluation vary in the way in which they measure benefits and the choice of which analysis to use for any particular service largely depends on which approach to benefit measurement is most practical.

Q: A new drug enables patients to live for 5 years rather than dying within

2 years. However, they live with a minor disability and a quality of life equal to 80% of a full healthy life year. But, if they do not receive the drug their quality of life for the 2 years they live is only 60% of a full healthy life year. How many QALYs are generated by the intervention?

A: 5 years of life at 0.8 QoL = 4 compared with 2 years of life at 0.6 QoL = 1.2. Therefore 4 − 1.2 = 2.8 QALYs generated.

Table 11.2 compares a range of different interventions in terms of their cost per QALY. Though all such data come with a health warning (costs vary), note how simple preventive interventions often compare favourably with highly specialised medical care.

In conclusion, priority-setting committees frequently use frameworks to advise organisations on the use of funds (*see* Figure 11.1). The aim overall is to provide a more robust decision than would be achieved through a less systematic approach, to ensure that resources are used cost-effectively and to enable improvement in the

TABLE 11.2 Cost per QALY for healthcare interventions

Intervention	£ / QALY
Cholesterol testing and diet therapy	220
GP advice to stop smoking	270
Neurosurgical intervention for subarachnoid haemorrhage	490
Antihypertensive treatment to prevent stroke	940
Pacemaker implantation	1100
Hip replacement	1180
Valve replacement for aortic stenosis	1410
Cholesterol testing and treatment	1480
Docetaxel (not paclitaxel) for recurrent metastatic breast cancer	1890
Coronary artery bypass graft (left main − vessel disease, severe angina)	2090
Kidney transplantation	4710
Breast cancer screening	5780
Heart transplantation	7840
Cholesterol testing and treatment incrementally	14150
Home haemodialysis	17260
Coronary artery bypass graft (single vessel disease, moderate angina)	18830
Hospital haemodialysis	21970
Interferon alpha-2b added to conventional treatment in multiple myeloma	55060
Neurosurgical intervention for malignant intracranial tumours	107780
Erythropoietin treatment for anaemia in dialysis patients	126290

	Intervention for A	Intervention for B	Intervention for C
Size/severity of the health problem			
Clinical effectiveness of intervention			
Cost implications			
Political considerations			
Acceptability of service to patients			
Equity and ethical considerations			
Total	*Stage 1 – Public Health*		

FIGURE 11.1 Prioritisation grid – for ranking different options

health of individuals and populations. In the last analysis, priority setting is an ethical process and needs to accommodate core values such as equity and patient choice.[4] Rationing decisions involve trade-offs and Figure 11.2 gives some of the dilemmas that are inevitably faced. Difficult choices involving public monies may be challenged at a local or national level, sometimes in courts of law. It is therefore essential that procedural justice underpins an open and transparent process in which the public, health professions, politicians and management all participate. Clinicians who combine technical and human understanding are central to the priority-setting process.

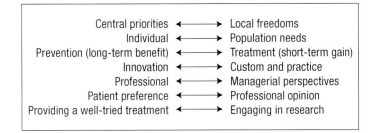

FIGURE 11.2 Dilemmas

REFERENCES

1 Griffiths S, Jewell T, Hope T. Setting priorities in health care. In: Pencheon D, Melzer D, Gray M, *et al.*, editors. *Oxford Handbook of Public Health Practice*. 2nd ed. Oxford: Oxford University Press; 2006. pp. 404–10.

2 Drummond M, Sculpher M, Torrance G, *et al. Methods for the Economic Evaluation of Health Care Programmes*. Oxford: Oxford University Press; 1997.

3 Phillips C, Thompson G. *What is a QALY?* London: Hayward Medical Communications; 1998.

4 Beauchamp T, Childress J. *Principles of Biomedical Ethics*. 3rd ed. New York: Oxford University Press; 1989.

CHAPTER 12

Scenarios

with Paul Cosford

SCENARIO 1: MANAGING CHANGE

This example is about achieving large-scale change across the healthcare system. There are times when clinical leaders become aware of a major source of harm to patients or people in the community, which should not be happening. This chapter looks at *Clostridium difficile* bacteria in an English region (the East of England) in some detail, drawing on one set of principles on how to achieve change. These principles are applicable to many different scenarios, and clinicians can use such principles to achieve improvements, whether at the level of the individual clinical team or within and among healthcare organisations.

The principles drawn on here are the eight steps to achieving change identified by John Kotter.[1] Many management theories sound like 'common sense', but using such a framework can ensure that the right steps are systematically worked through to achieve the change that is sought. The eight steps described by Kotter are:
1   create a sense of urgency
2   develop a vision for the future
3   develop a powerful 'guiding coalition'
4   communicate the vision
5   share the problem widely
6   empower people to act
7   identify short-term wins
8   institutionalise the change.

These events took place between 2007 and 2009 against a background of increasing rates of *Clostridium difficile* being reported in hospitals across the country. A small number of trusts appeared to have a particular problem. The report into *Clostridium difficile* at Maidstone and Tunbridge Wells had just been published, leading to major national media concerns and considerable publicity about safety in hospitals as a result. Information on rates of *Clostridium difficile* were available routinely for each hospital, but there were significant delays in the data being available for routine management use.

Step 1: Create a sense of urgency

This is vital to ensure that those who can make a difference believe that 'something must be done', that the current position is unacceptable and must be resolved. At this stage it is not necessary to know exactly *what* must be done. In some scenarios, the answers are complex and take time to develop. However, without the sense of urgency, sufficient effort will not be put into finding those answers and converting them into action.

In this example, the sense of urgency was initially created in an acute hospital that had had several deaths from *Clostridium difficile* in the previous quarter. Managers and clinicians were trying, thus far unsuccessfully, to prevent further cases. They were attracting media interest, with national newspapers wanting to report on numbers of deaths, and sending reporters to the hospital.

In addition to supporting the individual hospital in taking the actions needed to resolve their 'outbreak', more detail was sought about whether other hospitals in the region were affected. Since the routine nationally available data were some months in arrears, an agreement was reached with the hospitals to provide their provisional data directly to the strategic health authority, who could provide these data to all hospitals in the region in a timely and up-to-date manner. This led to the realisation that a similar problem was facing several acute hospitals in the region. At the same time, some acute hospitals had very low rates, suggesting that it is possible to have the problem under control.

If, as evidence clearly indicates, *Clostridium difficile* outbreaks are amenable to good infection and outbreak control measures, then large numbers of people were suffering avoidable harm, which could be reduced if appropriate action were taken. This needed a systematic approach across all the hospitals in the region, with clear leadership. Staff at the particular acute hospital concerned had no difficulty creating a sense of urgency – little concentrates efforts more than a tabloid journalist on the case of their next 'NHS scandal' story!

Q: What would you do to create this sense of urgency more widely?

Actions taken in this example included the following.
➤ Ensuring all National Health Service (NHS) leaders were aware of the position and saw this as a potential major reputational risk that needed addressing.
➤ Raising the issue of *Clostridium difficile* at every possible opportunity, with clinical and managerial leaders, and making sure they felt a responsibility for addressing the issue and reducing rates.
➤ Calculating an approximate number of deaths (about 10% of cases) that were likely to be resulting each month, and making sure that leaders of organisations were aware of this.
➤ Developing a new information system that allowed monitoring of up-to-date rates on a monthly basis and sharing this information widely. The position for all hospitals in the region was shared with the leaders of every hospital, both at meetings and remotely, so they could all see how they compared with others.
➤ Starting to report levels of *Clostridium difficile* in public NHS meetings.

Step 2: Develop a vision for the future

Sharing a vision of what may be possible is crucial to direct the efforts resulting from a sense of urgency into effective action.

> **Q:** What might help in this instance?

Within the region and elsewhere in England, a hospital that had previously had significant problems with *Clostridium difficile* and had resolved them was sought. This was to begin to give people leading and working in acute hospitals a sense of what is possible. To this end a hospital was identified with rates that had improved once all control measures were fully in place. Also identified were acute hospitals with the lowest rates, again to give an idea of what could be achieved.

In discussions with leaders across the region the idea was raised that it is possible to get very low rates in all hospitals. The argument was that, while most hospitals were implementing the majority of control measures most of the time, if they were all in place all of the time, infection rates would drop to very low levels. This vision was generally agreed, and led to the following.

➤ A public pledge to provide the safest healthcare in England and ensure 'no avoidable harm' to patients.

➤ An ambition to move from among the worst to the best rates of healthcare-associated infection in England.

➤ An aim for each hospital to have fewer than 12 cases of *Clostridium difficile* per month within a year. This was backed up by a financial incentive – national funding was provided to support reductions in healthcare-associated infection, which was doubled by the NHS regionally, but only on condition of the 12 cases per month challenge being achieved.

Step 3: Develop a powerful 'guiding coalition'

This is fundamental to Kotter's views as to how to achieve change in large organisations. This means developing a team of individuals with the requisite expertise from within the organisation who will explore the details of the situation, float ideas as to how the situation can be addressed and develop clear guidance as to how the organisation should respond in order to implement the change.

> **Q:** In this case, who should be involved and what should they be responsible for?

A regional Healthcare Associated Infection Taskforce was established, drawn from clinicians and managers from a variety of hospitals within the region. They included a range of disciplines (nurses, doctors, pharmacists), along with expert advisors from the Health Protection Agency, and those in management roles with expertise on implementation. The following three aspects were key to success.

1 Its responsibilities included identifying the evidence available on the nature of the problem and actions to implement change.

2 Their role was to advise managers and clinicians across the region from a group of expert and committed clinicians and managers about the necessary interventions and actions to reduce rates of *Clostridium difficile*.

3 Their recommendations were expected to be put into practice, and implementation audited. For example, they would advise on the use of antibiotics, appropriate hand-washing audits and what constitutes isolation for affected individuals. Hospitals were expected to implement their guidance.

Step 4: Communicate the vision

Kotter's next step is to ensure that the vision is effectively communicated, and the programme advised by the guiding coalition is made known by all who have any role in effecting the changes required.

Q: How would you have done this?

In the case of addressing *Clostridium difficile* this was achieved through a coordinated communications programme led by communications experts operating at both a regional and a local level. It included the following.

➤ Consistent communication of the current position at all meetings of managerial and clinical leaders, with sharing of up-to-date information on numbers of cases, recommendations of the taskforce and outcomes of audits of implementation.

➤ Ensuring that leaders of clinical teams were aware of what was expected of them and how their teams were performing relative to others.

➤ A specific newsletter, *HCAI News*, with up-to-date information, examples of best practice and individual stories of progress.

➤ Communication through workshops, conferences and other routes.

➤ Strategies and annual reports giving high profile to *Clostridium difficile*.

➤ Regular open communication with the media on the current position and actions being taken to address it.

Kotter's principle is that there needs to be a specific focus on getting the vision widely owned by all those who need to play a part in making it happen. In this case the vision was to have the lowest rates of healthcare-associated infection in England and fewer than 12 cases per month in every hospital within a year. The communications effort therefore initially focused on this vision, but in reality it also covered the next step of sharing the problem widely.

Step 5: Share the problem widely

This was achieved by:

➤ sharing information widely across all organisations so that each month leaders knew exactly their position relative to one another and to best practice

➤ within each organisation, staff at all levels being aware of the organisation's overall pattern of infection and their role in supporting changes to reduce infection rates.

The practical outcome was that everyone knew that they were part of a wider whole and had a practical contribution to make in reducing infection. It also unleashed the abilities of a far wider group of people to identify problems and to come up with solutions, which a simple top-down protocol-driven approach can never do. Two specific examples where this led to unexpected solutions follow.

1 A trust identifying that commodes were superficially extremely clean but that they had removable clip-on seats that concealed dirt and, therefore, risk of infection. This was then identified as a common problem in many hospitals, and led to a change to cleaning regimes as well as a search for new products that did not have this design problem.

2 A trust identifying that isolation rooms were ineffective because of plumbing deficiencies (i.e. no handbasins in each isolation room), which led to them providing 'stand-alone' washstands that enabled cleanliness within these rooms and improved infection control.

Step 6: Empower people to act

For change to be achieved across a whole system, people at all levels of an organisation must be able to identify problems and implement solutions within their sphere of influence. This needs to include managers, clinicians, other staff and patients. In the programme to reduce healthcare-associated infections this included, for example, the following.

➤ Communications campaigns aimed at patients, relatives and visitors supporting the concept that they should challenge staff who they did not see washing their hands before attending to them.

➤ The chief nurse in one hospital being empowered to open two isolation wards where people with *Clostridium difficile* infection would be cared for rather than in general wards (thus fulfilling the requirement for isolation). A medical director removing popular broad-spectrum antibiotics from wards within his hospital and instructing that they were only available for use with the express agreement of the hospital microbiologist.

➤ Developing a culture where staff felt empowered to challenge one another about hygiene (irrespective of hierarchy or profession).

Step 7: Identify short-term wins

To maintain the momentum required to change a whole system requires short-term successes to be made widely known. This is vital if people at all levels of the organisation are to maintain a belief that change is possible and that their efforts are worthwhile. It also gives kudos to those within the organisations that have achieved success and enables lessons to be learned.

In this example, the monthly monitoring of infection rates allowed those hospitals that achieved reductions to be identified quickly and that information shared rapidly through the various communication mechanisms already described. The experience also illustrated that, if all control mechanisms were in place for all patients all of the time, rates of infection fell precipitately. A good example was the hospital that identified that it had a problem early in 2007, and had significant tabloid media attention. When it successfully put in place the last of the control measures (isolation of affected patients) the rate of infection fell within a small number of weeks to among the lowest in the region (*see* Figure 12.1). This not only led to a strong sense of success for staff but also to a sense of what was achievable and within reach for all hospitals across the region.

Fundamental to this step is:

➤ identifying individual organisations where success is achieved early
➤ communicating widely their success and how they achieved it, sharing this information with other organisations, with staff and with the public.

Step 8: Institutionalise the change

This is critical to tackle the concern that a problem improves when it is being closely examined, but once the focus of attention moves elsewhere (as it inevitably will) the original problem reappears unless changes become a matter of routine practice. It is crucial to cement the changes that have been achieved as the new norm. At the point where all the actions needed have been implemented, the short-term change must become the long-term, sustained position for the organisation. In the case of *Clostridium difficile* this involved the following.

➤ Creating a cultural norm that low infection rates were the expected position for all NHS organisations in the region.
➤ Ongoing audits of expected practice in infection control and early intervention where any signs of relapse were identified.
➤ Setting expectations of low rates, and an ongoing reduction in rates, into the methods by which hospitals and clinicians are judged, and making the information on rates routinely available to the public.
➤ Embedding low infection rates in the regional patient safety programme.

Comment

This example has illustrated how the eight steps to change as described by Kotter can be used to achieve significant change to a major clinical safety issue across a whole healthcare system. While this might appear outside the influence of most individual doctors, it also indicates how health professionals working effectively together can have a major influence on the whole system and bring benefits to many patients. It also demonstrates that many of the factors needed are small-scale practical steps that, when taken together, lead to significant change.

SCENARIO 2: IMPROVING QUALITY

High-quality healthcare is about doing the right thing in the right way to the right person at the right time.[2] In other words, every patient who will benefit from an evidence-based, cost-effective treatment receives it whenever it is clinically indicated for them.

One common, often preventable, cause of morbidity and mortality related to

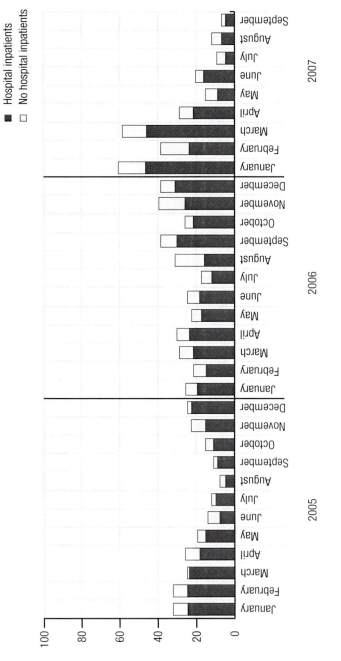

FIGURE 12.1 *Clostridium difficile* reports by specimen date month from hospital microbiology lab

healthcare is venous thromboembolism (VTE). There is good evidence available on how to prevent VTE but this is not systematically implemented everywhere, leading to unnecessary harm to patients. In fact, it is thought to be responsible for up to 10% of all deaths in hospitalised patients, and could account for about 25 000 deaths each year in England. A recent report from the Parliamentary Health Select Committee in England suggests that only 40% of at-risk patients receive appropriate prophylaxis.[3] Evidence from a typical English region suggests that VTE occurs in about 7.25 per 1000 high-risk patients who do not receive VTE prophylaxis and in 3.63 per 1000 high-risk patients who do. If 80% of patients were to receive prophylaxis this would prevent about 560 VTEs in that region, or about 5600 in England.[4]

So we have evidence that an effective preventative treatment for a relatively common condition is available, but is not being provided to everyone who should receive it. This situation has caused such concern that VTE has been the subject of various reports and of a clinical guideline by the National Institute for Health and Clinical Excellence. It has also been considered by the National Patient Safety Agency, and is included as a national requirement in quality measures within healthcare contracts between commissioners and providers of healthcare.

Despite this, at the time of writing there is still a long way to go before everyone who will benefit gets this preventive treatment. The question for clinical leaders in this scenario is how to take these recognised national priorities and ensure their systematic implementation at a local level, in particular in the hospitals and clinical teams within which the clinical leader operates.

This is another example where Kotter's eight steps to achieve change can be applied; this time at the level of a clinical team. Suppose that you are a junior doctor in a clinical team within an acute hospital, where the need for systematic approaches to VTE prevention has been recognised, and the clinical director has asked you to support her in introducing a programme to ensure every patient receives preventive treatment whenever it is appropriate. Work through the following questions before reading some suggested answers.

Q: How would you create a sense of urgency?

➤ Identify how many people cared for by your team are at risk each year, and the difference in numbers of people who will suffer from VTE if they all get appropriate treatment compared with the current level of prophylaxis. Bring this to the attention of your clinical director, and work with them to ensure all clinical and managerial staff within your team are aware of the potential harm that can be avoided.

➤ Seek support from the trust's communications team to publicise this to staff and to patients through newsletters, staff communications and other means.

➤ Prepare a poster with this information and display it prominently on the walls of wards, staff areas and other appropriate places.

Q: What would your vision be for the future?

That no patient cared for by your team should suffer avoidable harm as a result of VTE.

Q: Who would you include in your 'powerful guiding coalition'?

➤ Experts on VTE including a haematologist and specialist nurse.
➤ Clinical staff who deal with patients along the 'patient pathway' – for example, from A&E, the wards and operating theatres.
➤ Communications lead from the trust.
➤ A pharmacist who can advise on systems to ensure systematic prescribing to all appropriate patients.
➤ Clinical governance manager.

Q: How would you communicate your vision so it is widely shared within your clinical team

Raise the issue at clinical team meetings to gain their opinion on your proposed vision. When the vision is agreed to, have this written at the top of admission notes, in poster form on the walls of consulting rooms and wards and identified in electronic notes.

Q: How would you share the problem widely – so that everyone who needs to play a part understands their role?

Ensure that you have identified all the points during the patient's contact with the hospital and with your team when the need for prevention of VTE needs to be considered and assessed. Seek support from the trust's communications team to publicise the nature of the problem (as per first question) and activities that are taking place to address them.

Q: How would you empower these individuals to act, designing their own solutions where appropriate?

Run a competition to come up with the most effective way to stimulate change in practice at all stages of the patient's contact with the services at the trust. Run a communications campaign with patients to encourage them to ask doctors and nurses whether they have been assessed for their risk of clots.

Q: What do you think the short-term wins might be, and how would you identify and communicate them?

Talk with your clinical director to identify a ward or a hospital that has had a significant problem in the past and that has managed to ensure systematic application of best evidence since. Also, identify a step in the pathway that needs to change (e.g. a systematic decision aid to prompt assessment and appropriate prescribing on admission of the patient), audit its implementation and publicise widely those wards where implementation is most successful, indicating what can be achieved.

Q: How would you institutionalise the changes?

Draw up systematic decision aids that prompt assessment and appropriate prescribing as an automatic part of the admissions process. Confirm by regular audit that it is ensuring that all (or an agreed challenging target, e.g. at least 95%) appropriate patients are receiving thromboprophylaxis and seek support from the clinical governance or quality managers to report routinely the outcomes of the audit to the clinical directorate's management team and the trust board.

Comment
These examples illustrate the use of one widely quoted framework to support change; there are others. They can, of course, be applied to thinking about local as well as NHS-wide change.

SCENARIO 3: MEDICAL ERROR
You are a GP who is involved in the management of an out-of-hours primary care service. You are contacted one Sunday afternoon by the on-call manager of the ambulance service, who tells you that on the previous evening they were called to the home of a 68-year-old man whom they found unconscious, with signs of severe opiate overdose. Despite administration of naloxone, the patient died before the ambulance reached the local accident and emergency department.

At the time of the call the patient's wife informed the ambulance staff that he had renal colic and it was not unusual for him to need an injection to relieve the pain. She had called the out-of-hours service and suggested that this would be necessary. The locum doctor arrived, saw her husband, gave an injection and left. About 45 minutes later she went to see if her husband needed anything and found him unconscious, at which point she called the ambulance.

Q: What is your preliminary assessment of the severity of the situation?

The preliminary assessment is of a potentially very severe incident leading to death. There is insufficient information to be certain at this stage. However, there is enough to suggest at least the possibility of the out-of-hours doctor gave an injection of excessive opiate. If so, this may have been the cause of the death of the patient.

Q: What actions would you take immediately?

Immediate actions would be to determine which doctor was involved, to immediately call them to the service base and seek information from them about what treatment had been provided. Apart from the fact that the doctor will be the best source of information, you also want to make an assessment as to whether to stop them working while the incident is being investigated.

Q: What further information would you seek?

The medical records of the visit and of the patient if available, the log book in respect of controlled drug administration to determine what had been used and what other visits the doctor had made that weekend. These are useful sources of further information that should be immediately available. You are also wondering whether, if a serious prescribing error has been made, you will need to check the condition of other patients seen by the same doctor.

In terms of further actions, you have discovered that this was indeed a serious opiate drug administration error, in which the patient had been given 100 mg diamorphine intramuscularly. The GP concerned was a locum, had never practised in the United Kingdom before and was not used to using diamorphine (it is unavailable in his country of usual practice). It had been given from a 100 mg vial in the on-call bag, that vial being available for syringe drivers used in palliative care.

Q: What actions do you take in respect of the individual GP?

This is clearly a very difficult case, where the death will be the subject of a coroner's inquest and a police investigation. While mistakes do occur in medical practice with tragic consequences, and it is vital that clinicians are dealt with sensitively and not blamed inappropriately when mistakes happen, this is an extreme case where basic knowledge and competence appear to be in question. Your responsibility under the General Medical Council guidance for doctors is to comply with any police investigation, but also to ensure that the public are protected from any harm. In such an extreme case as this, you are likely to judge that there is a risk to patient safety if this particular doctor continues to practise unsupervised, and there needs to be a full investigation into the case and the doctor's competence. The appropriate actions are therefore:

1   To suspend the doctor from providing the out-of-hours GP service pending a full investigation.
2   To notify the General Medical Council so they can consider whether to act to restrict the doctor's practice in the United Kingdom (they can call an 'interim orders panel' within a few days, which can, if necessary, suspend the doctor's registration).
3   To request a 'professional alert letter'. This is a system whereby, if there is a significant risk to patients from an individual healthcare practitioner, a letter can be circulated to all NHS and private healthcare organisations indicating that, should the individual seek work with them, they should make contact with a specific individual at the original employing organisation to discuss concerns. At the time of writing it is requested from the strategic health authority. In future it is likely to be from the NHS Commissioning Board.

Q: Is there anything you wish to do in respect of other patients the GP has treated?

In view of the extreme nature of the error and its consequences, you should ensure an immediate medical review of all other patients seen by the GP over the weekend. This is an example of a 'look-back' exercise, where an identified error suggests other patients may be at risk of a similar error. They involve systematically identifying the patients who may have suffered harm, and providing an appropriate reassessment or information depending on the nature of the case. Judgements about whether a look back is required are often difficult and consultation is frequently required with national experts before deciding. In this case, however, there would be an immediate benefit to any patients who may have been erroneously treated, and therefore a look-back exercise is definitely required to ensure patient safety.

Q: Are there other aspects of this case you would want to make sure are fully explored?

These deal with whether systems should have been in place that would have made the error less likely, or whether existing systems are inadequate to ensure patient safety. They include the following.

➤ Availability of diamorphine in 100 mg vials. If only the small-dose vials suitable for intra-muscular injection were available this error may have been less likely. You therefore need to gain advice as to whether it is appropriate that 100 mg vials are available in out-of-hours on-call bags, and ensure action is taken to remove them if not. In this case, guidance from the National Patient Safety Agency had previously required a risk assessment of the availability of high-dose opiates and you will wish to ensure such a risk assessment has taken place in this service.

➤ The fact that a doctor not experienced in using diamorphine was practising as a locum out-of-hours GP raises issues about how people are deemed to be qualified to act as GPs and international agreements on mutual recognition of qualifications. These are not for you to sort out as a local GP, but it is your responsibility to ensure that these issues are raised with the appropriate authorities – for example, the medical director of the primary care trust or the regional director of public health.

Comment

This case achieved significant national publicity and a more detailed account of what happened and the lessons to be learned is in Cosford and Thomas 2010.[5] While such extreme cases are rare, the principles apply more widely.

SCENARIO 4: RISK MANAGEMENT

Eighty-one-year-old Mrs Irene P is admitted to hospital under the geriatricians with a chest infection. Early in the morning on the third day of her stay, she slips and falls on her way to the toilet. Her son complains verbally to staff that his mother 'ought not to be allowed out of bed so soon unaccompanied'. She is shaken but uninjured.

Q: What, if anything, should be done at this stage?

An incident report form should be completed. This will detail exactly what happened and what action was taken in response. Incident reports are routinely collected to form the basis of incident reviews. Learning from such reviews should be disseminated across the organisation as appropriate.

Three days later, under similar circumstances, Mrs P falls again. She is found by night staff at the door to the toilets. This time she has sustained a laceration to her chin that requires two stitches. She makes a full recovery and leaves hospital but 1 week later a formal letter of complaint is received from her son. He praises the quality of nursing care his mother received but wants to know why nothing was done in response to his alert following her first fall. He also mentions that the small step down into the toilet area could be hazardous for older people.

Q: What further actions need to be undertaken now?

A formal complaint requires a formal response. A carefully worded letter in this case would need to thank the son for his letter, to acknowledge his concerns and any points made as appropriate before detailing actions taken in response. Most complainants are seeking little more than an apology with assurances that action will be taken to prevent the same thing happening again. A more combative approach, even when any fault is not being accepted by the staff concerned is rarely, if ever, appropriate.

Three months later in the early hours of the morning, James B, an 84-year-old also admitted with a chest infection, slips and falls on his way to the toilet. Unfortunately, he sustains a fracture of his right hip. Night staff note the dilapidated state of his slippers but can find no other cause for his fall. Two weeks later he dies suddenly. At post mortem the cause of death is identified to be a pulmonary embolus.

Q: What could and should have been done to prevent this event?

➤ Slips, trips and falls are one of the commonest events with which clinical managers have to deal. Guidance on how to prevent falls is likely to have been distributed already but the earlier incident should have prompted a review of the ward's practice.

➤ Preventive actions include attention to individual patients' risk factors (past history of syncopal episodes, cardiovascular disease, other neurological or musculoskeletal conditions impairing gait and balance, polypharmacy, visual difficulties, confusion as well as the state of footwear). Environmental factors include unnecessary carpeting, steps, low lighting, clear signage and so forth.

➤ The 'quality gap' is the difference between understanding the need for quality improvement systems and how they affect actual practice. In this instance, the processes of data collection and report writing were in place but reviews of actual practice were not happening. No risk profiling of patients or ward checks had been undertaken. These events prompted a thorough overhaul of operating procedures in the hospital.

Q: What do you understand by the term 'risk management'?

Recent years have seen growing awareness of the number of errors, incidents and near misses that happen in healthcare and their effect on the safety of patients.[6] The science of risk management has borrowed heavily from other industries such as aviation. Risk management involves consideration of the following components:

➤ *Risks to patients* – these can be minimised through compliance with statutory regulations and ensuring that systems are regularly reviewed and questioned – for example, by 'significant event analysis' and learning from complaints. Root cause analysis (RCA) is an approach to problem-solving predicated on the belief that problems are best solved by attempting to correct or eliminate root causes, as opposed to merely addressing the immediately obvious symptoms. By directing corrective measures at root causes, the likelihood of problem recurrence should be minimised. However, complete prevention of recurrence by a single intervention is not always possible and RCA is often an iterative process.

➤ *Risks to practitioners* – ensuring that clinicians are immunised against infectious diseases, work in a safe environment and are helped to keep up to date are important parts of quality assurance.

➤ *Risks to the organisation* – in addition to reducing risks to patients and practitioners, organisations need to reduce their own risks by ensuring high-quality employment practice (including locum procedures and reviews of individual and team performance), a safe environment (including estates and privacy) and well-designed policies on public involvement.

Comment

In addition to identifying, analysing and treating them, risks must be evaluated. What is the balance between potential benefits and adverse outcomes of managing these risks? Not all risks can be completely eliminated even in the aviation industry. However, risk management strategies have little purpose if they are not monitored and reviewed. Are we improving the right outcomes? The medical protection societies are valuable sources of guidance on how to avoid and manage significant events.

SCENARIO 5: PERSONAL MISCONDUCT

Day one. The Medical Staffing department receives a phone call from the Emergency Department at around 11.30 a.m. to say that they have just realised that one of their junior doctors has not reported to work or called in to explain their absence. The junior doctor was due to start their shift at 8.00 a.m. The trainee in question is contacted by Medical Staffing. She apologises saying that she is having problems finding a parking space and will be in by 1 p.m. She does not report for work that day, although this is not communicated to Medical Staffing for several days.

Q: What are your thoughts on events so far?

➤ The internal systems appear inadequate, as it has taken several hours to notice that someone is missing. It can be easy in a large busy clinical department for people to get 'lost' in the system. This may need to be reviewed in the interests of both patient safety and that of individual members of staff.

➤ It is not plausible that it will take 5 hours to find a parking space. This should not be accepted as an excuse and it should be agreed that someone will discuss this with the doctor concerned. Everyone is delayed on occasions, but dishonesty is not acceptable and should ring alarm bells.

➤ The clinical department should have informed Medical Staffing sooner that the junior doctor did not attend work. Problems do not go away if they are ignored.

One week later. The Emergency Department contact Medical Staffing to say that it transpires that non-attendance has occurred on three previous occasions. 'What are Medical Staffing going to do about it?'

Q: What should the Medical Staffing and Emergency departments do now?

➤ The Emergency Department staff are right to raise concerns. However, this concern is not simply Medical Staffing's problem: their role is to support and advise; the clinical department have to engage in tackling the problem.

➤ An urgent meeting should be arranged with the doctor to discuss the concerns. She must be offered the right to be accompanied. The meeting should be supportive. Prior to this, references (from the deanery, her medical school, etc.) should be checked to identify whether there have been any previous concerns reported.

➤ The doctor should also be referred to the Occupational Health department.

The following day the junior doctor is interviewed and says that she had called in sick to Medical Staffing on the three previous occasions. Medical Staffing have no record of any such calls. Upon further challenge she admits she had been unwell on all occasions, but had not called in sick as did not want to 'let the team down'. She is feeling very stressed, is overwhelmed by the responsibilities of being 'on-take' and hints at difficulties in her personal life. Separately, another junior doctor mentions to one of the nurses in the Emergency Department that the junior in question is often late and quite dishevelled; on one occasion he thought he smelled alcohol on her breath.

Q: What would you do?

➤ You need to take an urgent view on whether to exclude/restrict her practice while the concerns are investigated. A formal written warning at this stage may suffice.

➤ The National Clinical Assessment Service (NCAS)[7] and the deanery should be notified. Consideration must also be given to notifying the General Medical Council.

➤ If major concerns are substantiated, a programme of support and rehabilitation may be required.

A year later, following a period of absence, the same junior doctor was working the weekday 'late' shift in casualty. She requested pathology investigations on six individual patients via the trust IT system. The following day an incident form was received by the Risk Management department from Pathology highlighting concerns that the section of the request forms reserved for clinical details of six patients instead contained offensive/inappropriate comments relating to high-profile public figures. The name of the doctor making each request was clearly highlighted on each form.

Q: What would you do and who do you think needs to be involved?

➤ You should seek advice from Medical Staffing to arrange a formal meeting with the doctor concerned. Technically, this constitutes further personal misconduct.

➤ Invite the doctor in question to a formal meeting to discuss concerns. She has a right to representation and someone from Medical Staffing should also be present.

➤ All serious concerns regarding medical staff must be addressed by the requirements in *Maintaining High Professional Standards in the Modern NHS*, which is the disciplinary, capability and ill-health framework for medical and dental staff.[8]

➤ Inform the chief executive who is required to appoint a 'case manager'.

➤ The case manager must be the medical director or a delegate.

➤ Appoint a non-executive director (NED) as the 'designated member' to oversee the case.

➤ You may need a 'case investigator', which should be a consultant from an unrelated discipline.

➤ Discuss your proposed approach with NCAS, who will retain a record on their database.

➤ Seek agreement from the deanery regarding the proposed approach as this concerns a doctor in training.

➤ Discuss with the educational supervisor whether there are any other concerns.

➤ The IT department should amend the patient records to remove the offensive comments.

At the formal meeting the doctor admits the offence. She claims she is under signifi-cant stress and having difficulty sleeping. She also claims she is seriously demoralised after the last few weeks of working in A&E. She felt bullied and intimidated by nurs-ing staff regarding 4-hour waits. She wrote highlighting her concerns to senior trust managers several weeks ago, and has not even received an acknowledgement of the letter. She admits she recently defaulted from an appointment with her educational supervisor. She is due to leave the trust in 10 days' time, moving to a rotation in a different region.

Q: What do you do now?

➤ Check when she is next due to work and make a decision about whether she is fit to work.
➤ Refer her once more to Occupational Health.
➤ Respond to the concerns raised regarding A&E.
➤ You still need to discipline the doctor as her behaviour was unacceptable and unprofessional. Issue her with a formal warning.
➤ Require the doctor to write and apologise to all of the people inconvenienced and caused unnecessary work.
➤ Inform the deanery to which she is moving as the formal warning will still be 'live' at the time of her next rotation.

Comment
Sadly, cases of personal misconduct frequently have past histories, suggesting that their problems may be long-standing and that earlier intervention might have pre-empted later problems.[9] The key to appropriate management of this scenario is an established, systematic, transparent and defensible procedure.

REFERENCES
1 Kotter J. *Leading Change.* Cambridge, MA: Harvard Business School Press; 1996.
2 Muir Gray JA. *Evidence-based Health Care: how to make health policy and management deci-sions.* London: Churchill Livingstone; 1997.
3 House of Commons Health Committee. *The Prevention of Venous Thromboembolism in Hospitalised Patients.* 2nd Report of Session 2004–05. London: The Stationery Office; 2005.
4 *Annual Report of the Chief Medical Officer for England.* London: Department of Health; 2009.
5 Cosford P, Thomas J. Safer out of hours primary care. *BMJ.* 2010: **340**: c3194.
6 *An Organisation with a Memory.* London: Department of Health; 2000.
7 National Clinical Assessment Service (www.ncas.npsa.nhs.uk).
8 Department of Health. *Maintaining High Professional Standards in the Modern NHS.* HSC 2003/012. London: Department of Health; 2003.
9 Yates J, James D. Risk factors at medical school for subsequent professional misconduct: multicentre retrospective case-control study. *BMJ.* 2010; **340**: c2040.

SECTION III

Being a leader and manager

There is no right or wrong way to learn how to be a manager. As you will have gathered, management – like medicine – isn't an exact science. One high-profile medical manager defined a sense of humour after intelligence and listening skills as the three most crucial attributes for a successful clinician manager.[1]

Some doctors become full-time managers but most clinical leaders will argue for maintaining clinical practice part-time. This is not just a matter of professional security in the longer term, but because they bring a unique perspective to management from active clinical practice. There are well-known pitfalls for 'player-managers', notably a tendency to over-identify with their tribe. It is harder to be wholly objective. Much can usefully be gleaned from watching or talking with the local clinical leaders and managers within the organisations in which you start work. There is no faster track for understanding the local politics and context. The trusted mentor can be enormously valuable. However, there are also courses for those doctors making a firm commitment to management – details of key providers of these are included later in this section.

After all this, is there any evidence that being a medical manager matters? Dorgan and Van Reenen studied almost 1200 hospitals in the United States, Britain, Canada, France, Germany, Italy and Sweden, using techniques more commonly applied to identify excellence in manufacturing industry.[2] The hospitals with the best management practices also ranked best on a standardised measure of medical success: mortality rates among emergency patients experiencing heart attacks. Five characteristics were associated with the management of successful hospitals. One was competition – or at least the perception of having competitors. Bigger was better when it came to good management. Hospitals employing 1500 or more staff are better run than those employing more than 500, which, in turn, outperformed those with more than 100 staff. Care must be taken to place international comparisons in context but private ownership appeared to help hospitals score more highly. Good staff also need the freedom to exercise their own judgement: managers with the most autonomy fared best.

Interestingly, institutions that employ clinically qualified staff in management scored better than those that do not. Overall, Britain performs badly by this measure: in Sweden, 93% of hospital managers are former doctors, nurses or other clinical staff. In the United States, Canada and Germany, the proportion is 71%–74%. In France it is 64% and in Britain just 58%. More such studies are needed – and more such doctors.

REFERENCES

1 Chantler C. Be a manager. In: *How To Do It 3*. London: BMJ; 1990. pp. 30–9.
2 Dorgan S, Van Reenen J. How to save lives: five simple rules for running a first-class hospital. *The Economist*. 21 October 2010. Available at: www.economist.com/node/17306072 (accessed 21 January 2011).

CHAPTER 13

Developing your leadership competencies

The aim of this book has been to develop your competencies in:

➤ leading people
  — understanding the nature of leadership
➤ adopting an appropriate management style
  — analysing accurately your environmental circumstances
  — analysing accurately the needs of the people reporting to you and to whom you report
  — identifying your own preferred management style
  — adjusting your style to the needs of the situation.

The following are some suggestions for activities you could undertake over the coming weeks and months with the aid of your colleagues, your boss or a mentor to develop these competencies.

➤ Like other aspects of the managerial role, you cannot develop leadership skills purely by accumulating knowledge – you need experience of leadership responsibilities and to learn from that experience. Consider the degree to which your current role offers you the opportunity to act as a leader, and in what ways. You could discuss with your boss or mentor ways in which your role could be tailored to ensure that you gain experience of leadership in a variety of settings, for example:
  — chairing a committee
  — heading a project team
  — taking on responsibility for the direct management of staff if you have not already done so.
➤ How do you make sure that you learn as much as possible from this experience? Two things are particularly important. First, you need to review your experience systematically, ideally with the help of a third party such as

a tutor. Second, you need feedback on your performance – from your boss, colleagues and subordinates.

— Keep a personal learning diary, noting important lessons from your experiences. Which leadership styles worked best, in which situations? What were people's reactions to your leadership? How did you feel on each occasion? Which style was most comfortable for you? Keep the diary conscientiously, and be honest with yourself!

— Arrange to discuss your experiences on a regular basis with your boss/ mentor. They can challenge you and offer you fresh perspectives. Sometimes learning can be enhanced by undertaking a review while the experience, and the feelings associated with it, are fresh in your mind. If your boss or mentor is not available, grab a colleague and discuss your experience with him or her.

— You need to actively seek out feedback on your leadership performance, from whoever has experience of it. For example, you could arrange for a colleague to observe your performance as chair of a committee and give you feedback afterwards.

— You can learn from the behaviour of those who are acknowledged to be effective leaders. If you can identify such people in your organisation, you could arrange to 'shadow' them for a period of time, identifying the features of their approach that seem to be effective. You will need to have a structure for your observation; ask your mentor for advice on what you might look for.

— The observation and the giving and receiving of feedback will be useful processes in developing your leadership skills.

➤ Inspiring others through the medium of ideals and values is the most difficult aspect of leadership to develop. However, some of the following exercises may be useful.

— Observe leaders in your organisation. Do they convey a sense of mission to their staff? If so, how? What differences in approach can you detect between those who do and those who don't?

— What gets you excited about your work? What makes it worth doing? What makes it important to your organisation? Try to write this down in a short and punchy 'mission' statement. What about the way in which it works? Can you write down a few important values that you would wish to hold by? If you can be clear about these things, you stand a better chance of conveying them with clarity to other staff. Discuss the outcome with your mentor, your boss or your colleagues.

CHAPTER 14

Managing your team

Most of the people you deal with work in groups or teams. Membership of a team can exert quite remarkable influences over people's behaviour. As members of a group, people will reach decisions and take actions that, as individuals, they would never dream of. If you regard people only as individuals, then, as a manager, you are ignoring some of the most significant and powerful influences that determine how well, or badly, they will work. Managers must, therefore, be acutely aware of the nature of groups, of the impact that they can have on individuals and of how to manage working groups so as to get the best out of them. Your task, as it was with individuals, is to influence groups so that they apply their efforts to the attainment of organisational goals.

There is another reason why an understanding of groups is essential for managers. As John Adair has emphasised through his 'Three Circles Model' (*see* Figure 14.1), all managers have three interlocking functions: to get the task done, take care of the needs of individuals who are working on the task and to maintain the cohesion, morale and effectiveness of the working group.[1] We have looked in some detail at the first circle – ways of getting the job done (planning, resourcing, setting targets and standards, controlling). We have also looked at the second circle – ways of satisfying the needs of individuals (by understanding them, recognising their needs, providing them with the kind of leadership they need, motivating them by designing their work and providing them with appropriate rewards). In this chapter, we consider the third circle – ways of managing the team so that it can work to optimum effect.

TEAM EFFECTIVENESS

Membership of groups satisfies important needs in individuals. Being a member of a group exerts powerful forces on the way a person behaves. An understanding of these forces can be very helpful to managers since they spend much of their working lives dealing with people in groups. Groups, it seems, are a natural and inevitable part of life.

➤ Managers create groups to get work done (task groups, project teams, sections, assembly lines, boards, committees).

➤ People form themselves naturally into groups to protect their interests (trade unions, professional associations, employers' federations, political parties, pressure groups).

➤ Most people satisfy their basic human need for belonging by being members of groups (informal groups, sports teams, clubs, working groups).

Q: You, as a manager, are almost certainly a member of at least one group in each of these categories, possibly several. List them.

Your managerial effectiveness is closely bound up with your ability to operate well as a member of a management group and to lead or manage your own working group. Most management courses, when they are offering guidance and advice on how to improve the effectiveness of groups, concentrate on those factors that can be changed in the short term – factors like the style of chairmanship (or leadership), the methods used for tackling problems and reaching decisions, the processes that could help the group to focus its attention on its task and that could smooth the interactions among the people in the group. But if groups are constructed for an inappropriate task, or with impossible constraints; if they are badly led or have ineffective procedures; if they have the wrong people, too little power or meet too infrequently, frustration will set in. The result will be an ineffective group.

Groups at work can be informal as well as formal. Informal groups are those that are not part of the formal organisation structure, and they may be led or dominated by people who have little or no formal authority within the organisation's structure. Nevertheless, such groups can be very powerful and very important for the way you carry out your managerial tasks. As we saw in Chapter 5, your effectiveness can be greatly affected by the norms of the group that you manage and by the extent to which you can influence them. Conflict among groups appears to be natural (us and them). Conflict can be beneficial when it leads to greater group cohesiveness and a stronger will to achieve. On the other hand, conflict between management groups and worker groups, which some people argue is inevitable, can be destructive.

Q: Are groups likely to produce *fewer or more* ideas than the individual members working separately? Are groups likely to produce *better or poorer* decisions than the individual members would take? Do groups take less *risky or riskier* decisions than the individual members would take? For the highest all-round involvement, is the optimum size of a group 3–5, 5–7, 7–9, 9–12 or over 12 people?

A: Groups are likely to produce *more* ideas than the individual members working separately. Groups are likely to produce *better, riskier* decisions than the individual members would take. For the highest all-round involvement, the optimum size of a group for most purposes is 5–7.

EXERCISE A

First select a group with which you work. Preferably, it should be a group that you lead or of which you are a member. Write the name of the group and its main purpose(s).

Name of group: _____

Purpose(s): _____

Group effectiveness is frequently related to the stage of development a group has reached. With reference to the stages in group development (Figure 5.2, p. 38), assess the stage your group has reached.

Stage of development reached: _____

As a basis for diagnosing possible faults in your group, and for prescribing possible solutions, consider the following questions.
- Is the group appropriately constituted to perform its task?
- Is it of a suitable size?
- Do the members have suitable characteristics?
- Are they sufficiently compatible for the complexity of the task?
- Are they clear what the task is?
- Is it a worthwhile task?
- Do they feel strong commitment towards it?
- Are they appropriately led?
- Does the group have a high enough status?

Against each heading in Table 14.1, mark your assessment of whether you feel that the present state of affairs is satisfactory or unsatisfactory for the purpose of the group. Where the present position is unsatisfactory, mark the right-hand column to show what needs doing to improve matters.

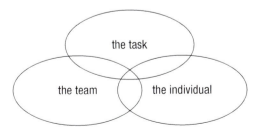

FIGURE 14.1 Adair's Three Circles Model

TABLE 14.1 Rating your group's effectiveness

Determinants of group effectiveness	Satisfactory	Unsatisfactory	What needs to be done
The givens			
The group			
Size			
Member characteristics			
Individual objectives and roles			
Stage of development			
The task			
The nature of the task			
The criteria for effectiveness			
Salience (importance) of the task			
Clarity of the task			
The environment			
Norms and expectations			
Leader position			
Intergroup relations			
The physical location			
The intervening factors			
Leadership style			
Process and procedures			
Task functions			
Maintenance functions			
Interaction pattern			
Motivation			

TEAM ROLES

Meredith Belbin and colleagues have undertaken much valuable work on the composition and functioning of management teams.[2] A team role is defined as a tendency to behave, contribute and interrelate with others in a particular way. They note the many roles that members can fulfil, and have shown how certain kinds of personality (extrovert/introvert, anxious/calm, etc.) tend to adopt certain roles consistently. They have given rather incongruous names to each of the roles. In addition to chair, these include the following.

➤ The *Plant* is the creative person with a fluent mind and divergent thinking who creates the new ideas.

➤ The *Shaper* is always looking for patterns in the team's discussions in an effort to unite ideas and push the team towards a decision and action.

➤ The *Monitor Evaluator* displays analytical thinking that enables him or her to access accurately the feasibility of proposed lines of thinking.

➤ The *Coordinator* has a capacity for converting decisions into practical lines of action and delegating tasks.

➤ The *Resource Investigator* has outside contacts and information and the ability to stimulate the team and preserve it from stagnation.

➤ The *Implementer* is disciplined, reliable and efficient in getting things done.

➤ The *Teamworker* offers support and help to individual members and builds up the social character and effectiveness of the group.

➤ The *Completer Finisher* galvanises the team into action and helps them to overcome the things that may go wrong or have already gone wrong.

➤ The *Specialist* is self-reliant, single-minded and with valuable in-depth knowledge; this was the last role to emerge and note that specialists have a weakness for focusing narrowly on their subject of choice and prioritising this over other team objectives – does that sound familiar?

They suggest five principles for establishing and integrating a management team.

1 Members of a management team can contribute to the team in two quite distinct roles: their professional role (medical, nursing, etc.) and their team role, as described in the previous list.

2 The effectiveness of a team will depend on the extent to which its members correctly recognise and adjust themselves to the relative strengths within the team, both in professional roles and in team roles.

3 Each team needs a balance of team roles. The optimum balance will be determined by its objectives.

4 Personal characteristics of individual members fit well for some roles and limit their ability to succeed in others.

5 Only when a team has a balance of team roles, represented by suitable people, can it deploy its technical resources to best advantage.

EXERCISE B

Consider the most important management team of which you are a member. Identify among your colleagues the individuals who best fulfil the roles described by Belbin.

Plant: _____

Shaper: _____

Monitor Evaluator: _____

Coordinator: _____

Resource Investigator: _____

Implementer: _____

Teamworker: _____

Completer Finisher: _____

Specialist: _____

Which role do you normally fill? _____

Are there any significant gaps in the composition of your team? Yes/No

In conclusion, anyone seeking a quick-fix solution that will instantly transform his or her group or team into a highly effective unit is likely to be disappointed, but such experimental work at least points the way to certain guidelines. Reflecting on your own work environment will best help you decide which of the many frameworks we have touched on in this book are likely to be of enduring value for you.

REFERENCES

1 Adair J. *Effective Leadership: a modern guide to developing leadership skills*. London: Pan; 1988.
2 Belbin RM. *Management Teams: why they succeed or fail*. 2nd ed. London: Butterworth Heinemann; 2004.

CHAPTER 15

Training for clinical leadership

These days the National Health Service (NHS), like other public services, is in a constant state of modernisation and reform. The challenge of encouraging clinicians into leadership roles is widely recognised but all health professionals need to understand the nature of change management. Doctors who don't, for example, understand how to influence policies within their workplace can rapidly become frustrated. The aim of this final chapter is to get you thinking about where you go next. How can you advance your professional development in these areas?

THE MEDICAL LEADERSHIP COMPETENCY FRAMEWORK

One possible starting point is the Medical Leadership Competency Framework (MLCF), which has been jointly developed by the Academy of Medical Royal Colleges and the NHS Institute for Innovation and Improvement. The MLCF describes the leadership competences doctors need in order to become more actively involved in the planning, delivery and transformation of health services.[1] It can be used to:
➤ highlight individual strengths and development areas through self-assessment and structured feedback from colleagues
➤ help with personal development planning and career progression.

The MLCF is built on the concept of shared leadership, where leadership is not restricted to those who hold designated leadership roles, and where there is a shared sense of responsibility for the success of the organisation and its services. 'Acts of leadership can come from anyone in the organisation, as appropriate at different times, and are focused on the achievement of the group rather than of an individual. Therefore shared leadership actively supports effective teamwork'.[1]

The MLCF evolved from a comprehensive review of the literature and an exhaustive analysis of other frameworks. It comprises the five domains shown in Figure 15.1. Each domain has four subsections corresponding to four competences to be attained, and each of these is further subdivided. Overviews of each domain are

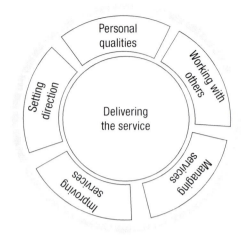

FIGURE 15.1 The five domains of the MLCF

shown in Box 15.1. The guidance provides a description of the knowledge, skills and attitudes and behaviours required for each subsection (*see* Figure 15.2). Following the individual domains, the guidance offers suggestions for appropriate learning and development activities to be undertaken throughout your training. A few examples are shown in Box 15.3.

BOX 15.1 Overviews of MLCF domains

Demonstrating personal qualities
Developing self-awareness by being aware of their own values, strengths and abilities to deliver high standards of care. This requires doctors to demonstrate competence in the following areas.
- Developing self-awareness by being aware of their values, principles and assumptions, and by being able to learn from experiences.
- Managing themselves while taking account of the needs and priorities of others.
- Continuing personal development by learning through participating in continuing professional development and from experience and feedback.
- Acting with integrity by behaving in an open, honest and ethical manner.

Working with others
Doctors show leadership by working with others in teams and networks to deliver and improve services. This requires doctors to demonstrate competence in the following areas.
- *Developing networks* by working in partnership with patients, carers, service users and their representatives, and colleagues within and across systems to deliver and improve services.
- *Building and maintaining relationships* by listening, supporting others, gaining trust and showing understanding.

- *Encouraging contribution* by creating an environment where others have the opportunity to contribute.
- *Working within teams* to deliver and improve services.

Managing services
Doctors showing effective leadership are focused on the success of the organisation(s) in which they work. This requires doctors to demonstrate competence in the following areas.
- Planning by actively contributing to plans to achieve service goals.
- *Managing resources* by knowing what resources are available and using their influence to ensure that resources are used and safely, and reflect the diversity of needs.
- *Managing people* by providing direction, reviewing performance, motivating others and promoting equality and diversity.
- *Managing performance* by holding themselves and others accountable for service outcomes.

Improving services
Doctors showing effective leadership make a real difference to people's health by delivering high-quality services and by developing improvements to service. This requires doctors to demonstrate competence in the following areas.
- *Ensuring patient safety* by assessing and managing risk to patients associated with service developments, balancing economic consideration with the need for patient safety.
- *Critically evaluating* by being able to think analytically, conceptually and to identify where services can be improved, working individually or as part of a team.
- *Encouraging improvement and innovation* by creating a climate of continuous service improvement.
- *Facilitating transformation* by actively contributing to change processes that lead to improving healthcare.

Setting direction
Doctors showing effective leadership contribute to the strategy and aspirations of the organisation and act in a manner consistent with its values. This requires doctors to demonstrate competence in the following areas.
- *Identifying the contexts for change* by being aware of the range of factors being taken into account.
- *Applying knowledge and evidence* by gathering information to produce an evidence-based challenge to systems and processes in order to identify opportunities for service improvements.
- *Making decisions* using their values, and the evidence, to make good decisions.
- *Evaluating impact* by measuring and evaluating outcomes, taking corrective action where necessary and by being held to account for their decisions.

3.1 Planning

Competence

1. Support plans for clinical services that are part of the strategy for the wider healthcare system
2. Gather feedback from patients, service users and colleagues to help develop plans
3. Contribute their expertise to planning processes
4. Appraise options in terms of benefits and risks

In the context of leadership and management activities, the following should be acquired by the end of undergraduate training in order to meet each specific competency:

Knowledge
Demonstrate knowledge of:

- Current NHS strategy
- Steps involved in planning change
- How to use pilots and trials as part of the planning process

Skills
Demonstrate the ability to:

- Select a quality improvement project and justify choice
- Set achievable project outcomes
- Work to project time lines

Attitudes and behaviours
Demonstrate:

- A systematic and organised approach
- Commitment to take the views of patients and service users into account
- Willingness to seek out and consider alternative approaches

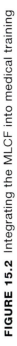

3.2 Managing resources

Competence

1. Accurately identify the appropriate type and level of resources required to deliver safe and effective services
2. Ensure services are delivered within allocated resources
3. Minimise waste
4. Take action when resources are not being used efficiently and effectively

In the context of leadership and management activities, the following should be acquired by the end of undergraduate training in order to meet each specific competency:

Knowledge

Demonstrate knowledge of:

- How resource is allocated in the NHS
- How resources are deployed within a service
- How extra resources can be brought into an organisation through bids and innovation

Skills

Demonstrate the ability to:

- Consider resource issues when:
  - discussing healthcare services and priorities
  - undertaking audits or service improvement exercises
- Formulate ideas for improving cost-effectiveness within a service

Attitudes and behaviours

Demonstrate:

- An awareness of funding constraints and need for cost-effectiveness
- A commitment to use NHS money effectively and minimise waste
- Readiness to challenge ineffective use of resources

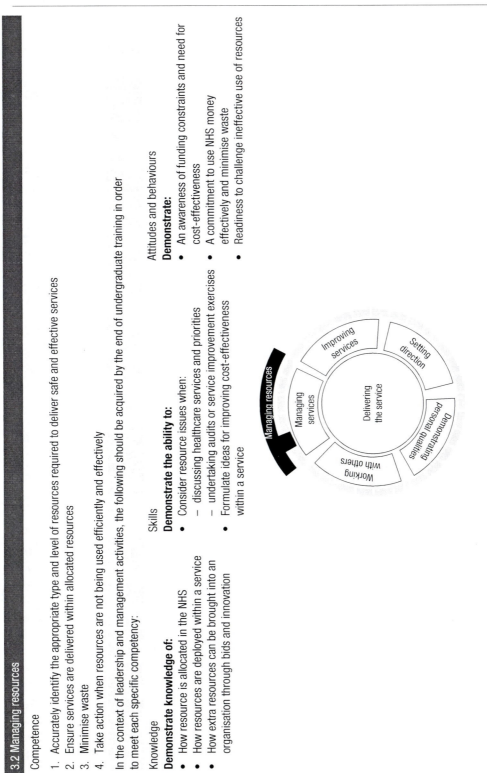

FIGURE 15.2 Integrating the MLCF into medical training

FURTHER TRAINING OPPORTUNITIES

For those of you interested in specific training, the options are legion. Some more business-minded doctors may undertake master's degrees in business administration (MBAs) or formal management diplomas. Many universities offer distance learning or part-time courses to run alongside the 'day job'.

There are numerous medical management development programmes in operation across the United Kingdom. Some of the best-known providers are detailed here but this list is not comprehensive.

The King's Fund – better known as a leading health policy 'think tank'. The Fund has long provided a variety of development programmes for managers in the NHS. Many of these are aimed at doctors taking on leadership roles. In addition to short courses, these are often based on learning sets that allow for learning in service (www. kingsfund.org.uk).

Health Services Management Centre – part of the School of Policy at the University of Birmingham, the HSMC is one of the leading centres specialising in policy, development, education and research in health- and social care services in the United Kingdom (www.hsmc.bham.ac.uk).

BOX 15.2 The Medical Leadership Pilot Programme

This runs alongside the current NHS Management Training Scheme and is delivered by HSMC, in partnership with the University of Manchester and The King's Fund. The pilot has provided a unique opportunity for NHS management trainees and NHS doctors in training to develop as leaders alongside one another. The pilot has demonstrated how working together can increase understanding of various clinical and managerial roles. It aims to foster relationships and networks that go on beyond the life of the programme.

British Medical Journal – the BMJ Group offers a number of online modules and events to assist doctors in their continuing professional development. The Clinical Leadership Programme provides postgraduate qualifications in clinical leadership for healthcare professionals. The programme has been developed by BMJ Learning in collaboration with the Open University Business School's Centre for Professional Learning and Development (www.bmj.com).

British Association of Medical Managers – until recently, BAMM offered doctors seminars, training programmes, a repository of literature and other resources. In 2008 BAMMbino was established as a network to promote management among junior doctors, tomorrow's clinical leaders.

Institute of Healthcare Management – the IHM is the professional organisation for managers throughout healthcare. It promotes high standards of management and is developing its educational portfolio (www.ihm.org.uk).

Institute for Healthcare Improvement – the IHI is a US independent not-for-profit organisation helping to develop safe and effective healthcare throughout the world. The IHI's programmes and activities are designed to enable committed individuals and organisations to innovate, share knowledge and collaborate on improving healthcare. A range of online courses (IHI Open School) covering many aspects of quality improvement and leadership are freely accessible to students (www.ihi.org).

BOX 15.3 Sample scenarios for exploring different MLCF domains

Developing personal qualities
A student shares with her tutor a patient encounter that has left her feeling upset. The tutor suggests that she writes a reflective piece as part of her portfolio to explore this issue. This helps her to identify her emotional response and the factors behind this, as well as to consider the encounter from the patient's perspective. She undertakes reading around emotional intelligence and stress management, and agrees some personal learning goals with her tutor.

Managing services
While on placement at their local hospital, students C and L are invited to support the investigation into a patient complaint relating to a refusal by the organisation to prescribe an expensive drug. Working with managers in the hospital complaints department, the students review the letter of complaint, seek advice on the hospital policy for prescribing and how this relates to National Institute for Health and Clinical Excellence (NICE) guidelines, and discuss the case with members of the clinical team. They draft a letter of response to the patient and write a summary report that they present to their clinical supervisor and peers, highlighting the management issues that arose from this example.

A final thought. Many people have been falling out of love with the notion of the great leader in recent years. The idea of the leader as omnipotent parent, whose power derives from access to special realms of knowledge and experience, strikes some as infantilising.[2] James Surowiecki in *The Wisdom of Crowds* suggests that aggregations of individuals often make better decisions than single individuals alone.[3] The surgeon Atul Gawande puts it pithily: 'We've celebrated cowboys, but what we need is pit-crews . . . it's teams and organisations that make for great care, not just individuals.'[4] In other words, trying to create a cadre of medical leaders is not the whole solution. All doctors need to become managerially competent. We hope this book has helped you on the way.

REFERENCES

1 Academy of Medical Royal Colleges and Institute for Innovation and Improvement. *Medical Leadership Competency Framework: enhancing engagement in medical leadership*. 3rd ed. NHS Institute for Innovation and Improvement, University of Warwick; 2010.

2 Delamothe T. Don't take me to your leader. *BMJ*. 2010; **340**: c2675.

3 Surowiecki J. *The Wisdom of Crowds: why the many are smarter than the few and how collective wisdom shapes business, economies, societies and nations.* New York: Doubleday; 2004.

4 Gawande A. Healthcare needs a new kind of hero: an interview with Atul Gawande. Interviewed by G Morse. *Harv Bus Rev.* 2010; **88**(4): 60–1. Available at: http://hbr.org/web/2010/04/gawande (accessed 7 March 2011).

Theories of management

For over a century, people have been studying managers at work in an effort to distil the principles that underlie good management. From such studies have emerged several different schools of thought with different approaches to management. There is no need for you to have a detailed knowledge of each, but being familiar with these alternative approaches can provide you with a variety of perspectives on your work. They can also yield a better understanding of your job and thereby lead to more effective performance. Here, eight approaches to management are reviewed in roughly the same order as that in which they emerged on the management scene.

THE SCIENTIFIC APPROACH

Around the turn of the twentieth century, Frederick Taylor and others began trying to apply scientific methods to management rather than the rule-of-thumb approaches then current. In other words, they brought the skills of observation, quantification, analysis, experimentation and evaluation to management in place of the more traditional precedent, intuition, personal opinion and guesswork. Their work gave rise to an approach known as 'scientific management'.

Taylor advocated five basic principles for his approach:

1   Give responsibility of organisational work to managers.
2   Use scientific methods to assess the most efficient ways of doing work (by studying tasks and specifying in detail how work should be undertaken).
3   Select training of workers scientifically.
4   Monitor work performance by relating detailed job specifications to particular outcomes.
5   Undertake 'management by exception', where routine decision-making is handled at a lower level and exceptional cases are handled higher up the organisation.[1]

Taylor's concern was to improve efficiency. His quest was to find the fundamental principles of efficiency, and underlying his search was the belief that there was 'one best way' of doing any job. He insisted that it was management's task, using careful experimentation and observation, to identify the one best method and to develop standardised tools (even down to the shovels) for implementing it. Then they should select their workforce very carefully, choosing only first-class people, and train them to use only the best methods. In this way, production could be improved and costs reduced. Workers would share in the resulting benefits by being rewarded for a 'fair day's work', their assigned goals being carefully determined by stopwatch studies. Taylor acknowledged that this could lead to higher wage costs, but he argued that management should be concerned less with labour costs than with overall costs per unit, and that his methods would lead, through increased output, to a reduction in unit costs. To achieve increased output per worker, he called on management to improve working conditions and reduce physical effort and fatigue.

THE PROCESS APPROACH

The process approach to management owes much to Henri Fayol's thinking at the beginning of the twentieth century. Fayol focused attention on the things that a manager does, and wrote that to manage is 'to forecast and plan, to organise, to command, to coordinate and to control'.[2] A hundred years later, his analysis still forms the basis of one of the most frequently adopted views of management, so much so that it is often called the 'classical view'.

There have been numerous attempts to improve on what Fayol wrote. For example, the idea of a manager 'commanding' now has a strangely old-fashioned ring to it. It has often been replaced by words such as 'directing' or 'leading', although these, too, can sound dated in the modern world, with its concern for ideas of participative management and democracy. As a consequence the word 'motivating' is often preferred because it sounds less loaded.

Into this category fall numerous theories of strategic management. 'Management by objectives' (MBO) was first popularised by the economist Peter Drucker. He suggested that the objectives for an organisation should be defined for each individual working there, both managerial and other staff. These objectives should be the basis for assessing performance thereby aligning goals throughout the organisation. It can certainly be argued that an obvious weakness of the National Health Service (NHS) is that the disparate, often conflicting objectives of different staff working within it. Clear and shared statements of purpose provide the basis of the organisational mission statements that Drucker also championed. Associated with this approach is the acronym SMART, suggesting that objectives should be specific, measurable, achievable, realistic and time-bound.

Strategic management theories have given rise to numerous formulations commonly employed within health and social services. These include the SWOT analysis (of strengths, weaknesses, opportunities and threats).

Mintzberg identified three types of strategies: 'intended strategy', as conceived by senior managers; 'realised strategy', which is that actually undertaken; and 'emergent strategy', which is the pattern of actions that emerge as managers respond to changing external conditions.[3] Realised strategies may follow from intended or emergent ones. The main message is that strategy development is not the neat and rational approach that some managers like to imagine. Cultural, political and other non-rational factors shape strategies and their implementation.

THE HUMAN RELATIONS APPROACH

Although its origins can be traced back to the nineteenth century, the human relations approach developed strongly during the 1940s and thereafter, partly as a reaction against the seemingly impersonal features of the scientific approach, but mainly because research studies during the previous two decades had demonstrated the importance of good human relations and the influence of social factors on workers' motivation. These so-called Hawthorne studies are regarded as a milestone in the evolution of management ideas. An important observation made in these studies was that output and morale went up every time management varied its working conditions, regardless of whether the change was for better or worse. The inference drawn from this was that workers respond positively whenever management appears to be concerned with their working conditions. This important finding is now commonly referred to as the 'Hawthorne effect'.

Elton Mayo, who was associated with the Hawthorne studies, concluded that:

➤ people are basically motivated by social needs
➤ they satisfy their needs through social relationships at work, rather than through the work itself, which often holds little satisfaction
➤ the work-group exerts more influence on a worker than do the incentives and controls used by management
➤ supervisors are effective only to the extent that they can satisfy their subordinates' social needs.[4]

In the years following the Second World War, men like Rensis Likert and Douglas McGregor conducted further research into group behaviour and management styles.

Likert's studies seemed to show that departments with low efficiency tended to be managed by people who were job-centred – in other words, by managers and supervisors who regarded their main function as being to get the job done – and who viewed people as being just another resource provided for this purpose. Such managers tended to adopt the attitudes that stem naturally from Taylor's scientific management: 'keeping their subordinates busily engaged on prescribed work, done in a prescribed way, at a prescribed pace, determined by time standards.'[1] Such methods, it was noted, could achieve high productivity, but they tended to create very unfavourable attitudes towards the work and the management, often resulting in strikes and stoppages, as well as high wastage rates.

Likert's studies also seemed to show that, in contrast, work groups with the best performance were often managed by people with genuine concern for their subordinates' well-being.[5] Such employee-centred managers and supervisors appeared to regard people as people, not as just another resource. In addition, they were perceived as exercising a much looser form of control, but they compensated by setting very high performance targets and by motivating people to meet them.

THE QUANTITATIVE APPROACH

As the name implies, the quantitative approach lays prime emphasis on the use of quantitative techniques. This approach can be traced back to Taylor's scientific management. However, a more recent antecedent is to be found in operations research.

The quantitative approach has gained impetus both from the availability of computers capable of storing the data in management information systems and from the ability of such computers to manipulate the complex mathematical models that are used to stimulate business activities. Computers allow us to collect a great deal of information about an organisation's day-to-day activities. Sophisticated software programs allow such information to be pulled together, 'smoothed' to remove aberrations and displayed in boardrooms in readily assimilable formats such as pie charts and diagrams. Such programs assist short-term forecasting and thus allow optimum use of resources to be planned.

THE SYSTEMS APPROACH

Systems thinking developed concurrently with the quantitative approach, and emerged strongly during the 1960s and 1970s. It is an approach that emphasises the interrelatedness and interdependence of the parts and the way in which this contributes to the functioning of the whole. It is not unique to management thinking, having been applied to problems in many scientific fields, but it provides a helpful way of looking at many management problems, particularly those concerned with organisations.

When the systems approach is applied to organisations, it highlights the obvious point that if any part of a system is altered it is likely to have repercussions for the system as a whole – the magnitude of the repercussions depending on the nature of the change and the system affected. It follows that managers need to understand the way in which their own units or sections relate to other parts of the organisation and to the functioning of the organisation as a whole.

Every system and subsystem (unit or section) has a boundary that separates it from all the others. A closed system is one that functions entirely within its own boundary, and is unaffected by anything outside itself. Most systems, however, are open and are interrelated to others. The concept of boundaries is important to managers, for it is there that problems all too easily arise.

For a system to function effectively, resources such as materials, money, human resources and information must flow freely through the system. The flow may be affected by a variety of factors, which may be human as well as technical, and both are important subsystems that need to be given careful consideration.

THE ORGANISATIONAL BEHAVIOUR APPROACH

This developed from the human relations approach, and builds on the belief that in order to put strategies into action people must be encouraged to act in a way that produces the desired results. In line with the human relations approach, the organisational behaviour (OB) approach is concerned with people as individuals, their behaviour in groups, their individual motivations, their development within the organisation and their receptivity to new ideas and change.

However, in addition, the OB approach takes into account the organisational structures within which people work. Do the structures allow people to come together in the right groupings to perform a task or to make a decision, or do the barriers of division or department, or the hierarchical structure, or the complexity of the decision-making structures get in the way?

OB approaches remain pervasively influential. They seek to match an individual's aspirations as closely as possible with those of the organisation, so that what is good for the organisation is good for the individual. Managers cognisant of OB theories try to create an environment in which learning and personal development take place, and typically encourage staff training and coaching. This benefits individuals in terms of career development and the organisation in terms of the quality of workforce.

THE CONTINGENCY APPROACH

In essence, this approach takes the view that 'it all depends on circumstances'. Circumstances, as we well know, can be totally different from one situation to another, and the situational approach recognises that it is impossible to prescribe any single solution that will be best in all circumstances and situations. In contrast with Taylor, it claims there is no 'one best way'.

'Contingency theory' argues that the structure required is contingent on the circumstances. In other words, structures must be adapted to the circumstances. The theory suggests that an organisation will be more successful if it consciously adapts its structures and its administrative arrangements to the tasks that need to be done, the technology that is used, the expectations and needs of the people performing the tasks, the scale of the total operation, and the complexity and change it has to deal with in its environment. In some versions of this approach there is a flavour of natural selection, which suggests that those who do not adapt do not survive.

Large and complex organisations end up with different designs for different parts of themselves, because the circumstances differ in different parts of the organisation and call for different answers. Very much reflecting the views of the OB approach, contingency theory suggests that people with different needs and motivations need different forms of management structure if they are to function well. Thus, people with a high need for security, a low tolerance of ambiguity and a dislike of risk and chance tend to work best under a tight structure. Young, ambitious and skilled people tend to work better under a looser rein.

The nature of the job to be done has been seen by many writers as crucial to the structure. If the tasks are clear, short-term and unchanging, then the structure can be straightforward and the control mechanisms very simple. If the tasks are more diverse, they require more complex structures and more complicated organisations.

Within the NHS the concentration of patient care and services into larger units, so as to gain the benefits of economies of scale, has led to the creation of larger management and administrative hierarchies. However, within these hierarchies most units and departments are in the process of adapting to a variety of different circumstances – to meet different environmental influences, to take advantage of new technologies and to cope with changes in the scale of operation. There is invariably scope for flexibility within this overall framework.

MODERNIST APPROACHES

Systems thinking, referred to earlier, highlighted the importance of considering the interdependence of different organisations. Recent theories agree on flattening hierarchies, facilitating informal networks and promoting diversity. They question simple realist beliefs about the world and are underpinned by sociological and philosophical theories such as social constructivism, critical theory, phenomenology, postmodernism and complexity theory. We will touch on complexity theory and postmodernism briefly here but interested readers are referred to the Bibliography at the end of this appendix for more comprehensive introductions.

Complexity theory

The science of complexity is concerned with the behaviour of non-linear networks consisting of a large number of agents employing sets of rules to interact with the system. The classic example would be a flock of birds in flight. The complex adaptive system (CAS) tends to be highly distributed and decentralised. The overall behaviour of the system is a result of a huge number of decisions taken simultaneously by many different agents. Fundamental principles apply to CASs: self-organisation, productivity and independence, positive and negative feedback and the evolution of both the system and the environment.

Theorists have applied ideas from chaos theory to CAS to define three behaviour types: chaotic, stable and unchanging, and innovative verging on the edge of chaos. NHS managers may identify with the third of these. The application of complexity theory to organisations demands a mind shift from managers and acceptance that the long-term future operation of their organisation is inherently unpredictable. Long-term planning is therefore less valuable than continual transformation in the face of constantly emerging environmental circumstances. Again, this resonates with the experience of managers in an ever faster changing NHS.

The claim that the NHS and other organisations are complex adaptive systems governed by the mathematical laws of chaos may be appealing but is as yet unsupported by much evidence. The promotion of a more egalitarian and less controlling approach allowing organisational solutions to problems to emerge has much in common with the humanist theories discussed here. However, it remains to be seen whether complexity theory will become more than a fashionable fad.

Postmodern management

Some of the same suspicions surround the application of ideas of postmodernist philosophers such as Foucault and Derrida to management thinking. Postmodernism rejects the idea that knowledge represents an externally existing reality and that language provides value-free, objective descriptions of it. At one extreme, in this view if empirical approaches in management are no more than processes of professional self-justification, the promise is to get rid of management altogether. At the very least, small is beautiful in organisational terms.

Postmodern approaches seek to promote diversity rather than a shared organisational culture. Postmodernism does not offer concrete methods or approaches for managers but is against centralising tendencies and draws attention to the diversity of stakeholders that need to be involved in decision-making.

CONCLUSION

An essential contention in this book is that management and leadership in healthcare are in many ways unsuitable for rational objectivist and classical approaches. Yet, ironically, these remain a dominant paradigm and they have been reinforced by the market-oriented agenda of successive governments.

More mechanistic approaches to management based on rational planning retain enduring appeal. They work well when the tasks to be performed are straightforward and the environment is stable, when precision rather than discretion and judgement is at a premium, when the human cogs in the machine conform to routine roles. Some areas of healthcare work like this – for example, the operating theatre – but many do not.

The key weakness of such models is that their rule-based structures may make them rigid and inflexible, restraining creativity and innovation. Unfortunately, public sector organisations are often rated highly on bureaucratic, reactive and authoritarian measures and lowest on the accessible, empowering and innovative ones. At times of external turbulence, organisations as experienced by the managers within them often become more bureaucratic, reactive and authoritarian. We see this in times of financial hardship within the NHS. Many view the present trend to standardise and control healthcare through excessive target setting, audit and regulation, as resulting in services that are less sensitive for users and of poorer quality. Classical management approaches with clear visions, specific targets and accountability can devalue the human nature of health services. In contrast, newer management models seek to embrace the intrinsic uncertainty of health and social services.

REFERENCES

1 Taylor FW. *Scientific Management*. New York: Harper & Row; 1947.
2 Fayol H. *General and Industrial Management*. London: Pitman; 1949.
3 Mintzberg H. *The Nature of Managerial Work*. New York: Harper & Row; 1973.
4 Mayo E. *The Human Problems of Industrial Civilisation*. London: Macmillan; 1933.

5 Likert R. *The Human Organisation: its management and value*. New York: McGraw-Hill; 1967.

BIBLIOGRAPHY

There are numerous readable introductions to management theory. A short personal listing is included here. The writings of the most popular management theorists are (usually) accessible. Communication skills are, after all, one of their major selling points.

- Charles Handy. *Understanding Organisations*. London: Penguin; 1989. This classic text illuminates key managerial concepts and applies them to practical problems. His Irish roots are betrayed in a colourful writing style that has made his books bestsellers.
- John Lawler, Andy Bilson. *Social Work Management and Leadership: managing complexity with creativity*. London: Routledge; 2010. An excellent recent summary of the field covering more contemporary theories. Written for students of social care, the book is a useful resource for health sector managers also.
- Derek Pugh, David Hickson. *Writers on Organisations*. 5th ed. London: Penguin; 2007. An invaluable introduction to the ideas and arguments of leading writers on management.
- Peter Drucker. *The Practice of Management*. New York: HarperBusiness; 1954. The need to manage business by balancing a variety of goals, rather than subordinating an institution to a single value, and the concept of management by objectives form the core of this landmark publication. Drucker's writings were marked by a focus on relationships among human beings and how organisations can bring out the best in people.
- Peter Senge. *The Fifth Discipline: the art and practice of the learning organization*. New York: Doubleday; 1994. Senge's notion of the 'learning organisation', a dynamic system constantly adapting and improving, where people continually expand their capacity to create the results they desire, has been widely influential beyond the private sector.
- Donald Schon. *The Reflective Practitioner: how professionals think in action*. New York: Basic Books; 1984. Schon's writings extended key twentieth-century theories of education. Once a 'must-read' for medical teachers, this book examines the nature of truly reflective practice.

Management competencies

In the main, we have not taken a competency-based, checklist approach to our topic. We hope to have stimulated you to learn more about the complexity of management and leadership by pointing to the wide and fascinating range of theories and approaches that inform the field. This section provides a concessionary 'how-to' approach to some commonplace tasks.

TIME MANAGEMENT

How often do you find yourself running out of time? Weekly, daily, hourly? For many, it seems that there's just never enough time in the day to get everything done. When you know how to manage your time you gain control. Rather than busily working here, there and everywhere (and not getting much done anywhere), effective time management helps you to choose what to work on and when. This is essential if you're to maximise achievements.

The following time management quiz (p. 136) devised by MindTools, an online source of numerous management resources (www.mindtools.com/pages/article/newHTE_88.htm), may help you identify the aspects of time management that you need most help with. The results will point you to the specific tools you need to use to gain control of your time and start working efficiently.

For each question, tick the the column that most applies. Add up your score and check your result against the scoring table underneath.

As you answered the questions, you probably had some insight into areas where your time management could be improved. The following is a quick summary of the main areas of time management that were explored in the quiz.

Goal setting (questions 6, 10, 14, 15)

To start managing time effectively, you need to set goals. When you know where you're going, you can then figure out what exactly needs to be done, in what order.

Question	Not at all 1	Rarely 2	Sometimes 3	Often 4	Very Often 5
1 Are the tasks you work on during the day the ones with the highest priority?					
2 Do you find yourself completing tasks at the last minute, or asking for extensions?					
3 Do you set aside time for planning and scheduling?					
4 Do you know how much time you are spending on the various jobs you do?					
5 How often do you find yourself dealing with interruptions?					
6 Do you use goal-setting to decide what tasks and activities you should work on?					
7 Do you leave contingency time in your schedule to deal with 'the unexpected'?					
8 Do you know whether the tasks you are working on are of high, medium or low value?					
9 When you are given a new assignment, do you analyse it for importance and prioritise it accordingly?					
10 Are you stressed about deadlines and commitments?					
11 Do distractions often keep you from working on critical tasks?					
12 Do you find you have to take work home, in order to get it done?					
13 Do you prioritise your 'To Do' list or Action Program?					
14 Do you regularly confirm your priorities with your boss?					
15 Before you take on a task, do you check that the results will be worth the time put in?					

Total =

Score Interpretation

Score	Comment
46–75	You're managing your time very effectively! Still, check the sections below to see if there's anything you can tweak to make this even better.
31–45	You're good at some things, but there's room for improvement elsewhere. Focus on the serious issues below, and you'll most likely find that work becomes much less stressful.
15–30	The good news is that you've got a great opportunity to improve your effectiveness at work, and your long-term success. However, to realize this, you've got to improve your time management skills. Start below!

Without proper goal setting, you'll fritter your time away on a confusion of conflicting priorities. People tend to neglect goal setting because it requires time and effort. What they fail to consider is that a little time and effort put in now saves an enormous amount of time, effort and frustration in the future.

Prioritisation (questions 1, 4, 8, 9, 13, 14, 15)

Prioritising what needs to be done is especially important. Without it, you may work very hard, but you won't be achieving the results you desire because what you are working on is not of strategic importance.

Most people have a 'to-do' list of some sort. The problem with many of these lists is they are just a collection of things that need to get done. There is no rhyme or reason to the list and, because of this, the work they do is just as unstructured. So how do you work on to-do list tasks – top down, bottom up, easiest to hardest?

To work efficiently you need to work on the most important, highest value tasks. This way you won't get caught scrambling to get something critical done as the deadline approaches.

Managing interruptions (questions 5, 9, 11, 12)

Having a plan and knowing how to prioritise it is one thing. The next issue is knowing what to do to minimise the interruptions you face during your day. It is widely recognised that managers get very little uninterrupted time to work on their priority tasks. There are phone calls, information requests, questions from employees and a whole host of events that crop up unexpectedly. Some do need to be dealt with immediately, but others need to be managed.

However, some jobs need you to be available for people when they need help – interruption is a natural and necessary part of life. Here, do what you sensibly can to minimise it, but make sure you don't scare people away from interrupting you when they should.

Procrastination (questions 2, 10, 12)

'I'll get to it later' has led to the downfall of many a good employee. After too many 'laters' the work piles up so high that any task seems insurmountable. Procrastination is as tempting as it is deadly. The best way to beat it is to recognise that you do indeed procrastinate. Then you need to figure out why. Perhaps you are afraid of failing? (And some people are actually afraid of success!)

Once you know why you procrastinate then you can plan to get out of the habit. Reward yourself for getting jobs done, and remind yourself regularly of the horrible consequences of not doing those boring tasks!

Scheduling (questions 3, 7, 12)

Much of time management comes down to effective scheduling of your time. When you know what your goals and priorities are, you then need to know how to go about creating a schedule that keeps you on track, and protects you from stress.

This means understanding the factors that affect the time you have available for work. You not only have to schedule priority tasks, you have to leave room for interruptions, and contingency time for those unexpected events that otherwise wreak chaos with your schedule. By creating a robust schedule that reflects your priorities and well as supports your personal goals, you have a winning combination and one that will allow you to control your time and keep your life in balance.

Time management is an essential skill that helps you keep your work under control, at the same time that it helps you keep stress to a minimum. We would all love to have an extra couple of hours in every day. As that is impossible, we need to work smarter on things that have the highest priority, and then creating a schedule that reflects our work and personal priorities.

With this in place, we can work in a focused and effective way, and really start achieving those goals, dreams and ambitions we care so much about.

APPRAISAL: GIVING AND RECEIVING

Principles of appraisal

Appraisal for doctors is a professional process of constructive dialogue, in which the doctor being appraised has a formal, structured opportunity to reflect on their work and to consider how their effectiveness might be improved. The NHS (National Health Service) Appraisal Toolkit provides useful online resources for both appraisers and appraisees.[1]

Appraisal should be a positive process to give doctors feedback on their past performance, to chart their continuing progress and to identify development needs. It is also a forward-looking process, essential in identifying the developmental and educational needs of individuals. The primary aim of appraisal is to help doctors consolidate and improve on good performance. In doing so, it will identify areas where further development may be necessary or useful. It can help to identify reductions in performance at an early stage; and also to recognise factors that may lead to a reduced level of performance, such as ill health.[2]

BOX A2.1 Aims of appraisal

- Set out personal and professional development needs and agree plans for these to be met.
- Review regularly a doctor's work and performance, utilising relevant and appropriate comparative operational data from local, regional and national sources.
- Consider the doctor's contribution to the quality and improvement of services and priorities delivered locally.
- Optimise the use of skills and resources in seeking to achieve the delivery of general and personal medical services.
- Identify the need for adequate resources to enable any service objectives in the agreed job plan review to be met.
- Provide an opportunity for doctors to discuss and seek support for their participation in activities for the wider NHS.
- Utilise the annual appraisal process and associated documentation to meet the requirements for General Medical Council (GMC) revalidation against the seven headings of the GMC's *Good Medical Practice* document.

Appraisal will underpin continuing professional development and also provides doctors with an opportunity to demonstrate the evidence for revalidation. While appraisal is formative, revalidation is a summative process. Revalidation is a judgement as to whether a doctor can remain on the medical register, and the revalidation process will inform the GMC's decision (every 5 years) about whether or not to renew an individual's registration.

How appraisal works

Appraisal is personal; its purpose is to support the individual development of doctors. The process should:
➤ emphasise a positive and developmental approach
➤ be fair and effective
➤ be well informed
➤ show how patient care and working within NHS organisations can be improved
➤ have adequate preparation time, and be adequately prepared for by both appraiser and appraisee
➤ have a specific time set aside for the appraisal
➤ be undertaken at regular intervals with skill, professionalism and confidentiality
➤ be properly supported by the primary care trust (PCT) or trust.

The content of appraisal will be based on the core headings set out in the GMC's *Good Medical Practice* document, together with consideration of the doctor's contribution to meeting local patient needs. The GMC's core headings are:

➤ Good clinical care
➤ Maintaining good medical practice
➤ Relationships with patients
➤ Working with colleagues
➤ Teaching and training
➤ Probity
➤ Management activity
➤ Research
➤ Health.

Appraisal offers the chance to reflect on these issues with the skilled facilitation of a trained appraiser. Key principles underpinning the appraisal interview are that it should:
➤ be confidential
➤ find solutions with realistic goal setting
➤ be person-centred and participative
➤ be future-oriented
➤ be developmental and supportive
➤ promote learning through reflection.

Being appraised: the process

This is not just about an annual interview. As an appraisee, consider these stages of the process:
➤ consider priorities and contexts
➤ reflect on practice – review the past year
➤ choose which tools can help in this reflection/review
➤ apply the tools
➤ review the results
➤ complete appraisal questionnaire
➤ prepare written submission to appraiser
➤ appraisal interview
  — consider submission in the light of priorities and contexts
  — generate learning needs, and plan learning activities
  — generate agreed report
  — generate outline learning portfolio
➤ carry out learning plan, prepare for next appraisal.

Preparation for the appraisal is essentially an opportunity to reflect on and review your practice or hospital over the last year. This reflection and review is carried forward into the appraisal itself. The purpose of this is to:
➤ provide an opportunity to discuss your job, hopes, aspirations and plans
➤ chart progress and development
➤ reflect on performance
➤ discuss how personal plans fit with wider planning

- ➤ give and receive feedback that is honest, sensitive and respectful
- ➤ demonstrate the value of the individual
- ➤ produce solutions
- ➤ influence and contribute to the practice or hospital development plan and the PCT/trust local health plan
- ➤ review progress on portfolio development.

The doctor being appraised should prepare for the appraisal by identifying those issues that they wish to raise with the appraiser and prepare a proposed personal development plan (PDP). The appraisee should gather information about, and reflect upon, the following questions.

- ➤ Am I a good doctor?
- ➤ Am I up to date?
- ➤ Do I work well in a team?
- ➤ What resources and support do I need?
- ➤ How well am I meeting my personal, practice/hospital or PCT/trust objectives?
- ➤ What are my development needs?

The information and paperwork to be used in the appraisal discussion should be shared between the appraiser and the appraisee at least 2 weeks in advance to allow for adequate preparation for the discussion and validation of supporting information. The discussion should be based on accurate, relevant, up-to-date and available data. The appraisal discussion should be held in a comfortable work setting, free from interruptions and distractions such as phone calls and demands from other staff.

Different people prefer different methods of reflection. Some people will jot down notes while others may write more formally. Some people will talk things over with colleagues or with their partner, while others may sit and think, or go for a walk.

The formal part of the preparation for the appraisal is completion of the appraisal questionnaire. For some the process of completing this questionnaire will stimulate all the reflection required, others will need to use other methods of reflection before they fill in the questionnaire, or they may need to break off part way through. Prompts to reflection provided in the 'NHS Appraisal Toolkit' include:

- ➤ lists of local and national priorities
- ➤ review of critical incidents diaries / significant event logs
- ➤ review of audits
- ➤ review of practice report or practice professional development plan
- ➤ review of complaints or suggestions from patients
- ➤ review of prescribing data, referral data and other aspects of practice.

As a result of this reflection you may wish to gather some evidence by looking at the way you practice. This could involve peer (e.g. mentoring, direct observation) or multidisciplinary assessment (e.g. 360 degree initiatives, case discussion).

The appraisal should conclude by setting down in an action plan the agreements that have been reached about what each party is committed to doing. This should include the essentials of a PDP. The appraisal should identify individual needs that will be addressed through the PDP. The plan should also provide the basis for assessment of resource needs and clinical governance issues within a practice/ hospital.

The appraiser and appraisee will agree a written overview of the appraisal that should, as a minimum, include:

➤ a synopsis of achievement in the previous year
➤ objectives (an action plan) to be pursued by the appraisee over the next year
➤ actions expected of the PCT/trust to address needs in the local context or wider system
➤ the key elements of a PDP for the appraisee
➤ a standard summary of the appraisal as recommended by the GMC for the individual's revalidation folder
➤ a joint declaration that the appraisal has been carried out properly.

The key points of the discussion and outcome must be fully documented and copies held by the appraiser and appraisee. Both parties must complete and sign the appraisal summary statement and send a copy, in confidence, to the senior clinican/ clinical governance lead and chief executive of the PCT/trust. All records will be held on a secure basis and access/use must comply fully with the requirements of the Data Protection Act.

Where significant problems have been identified, observations about further operational, financial or premises help required by the GP would be sent to the PCT/ trust chief executive. The detailed content of the appraisal itself should be confidential between the doctor and the appraiser.

Appraising a colleague: the process

Now think about how you would approach the appraisal of a colleague – whether medical or non-medical. What principles underlie your approach? How should you prepare for, conduct and conclude an appraisal?

For the appraisal to be effective, the interaction between the appraiser and the appraisee needs to be as open as possible. The giving of feedback (by the appraiser) and the disclosure of areas of concern (by the appraisee) are related processes, both of which rely on trust. To nurture this trust there must be clarity about the scope of confidentiality in the appraisal.

Giving information

Information giving is more likely to be successful if the speaker and listener are on the same wavelength, if the information is broken down into manageable chunks and if the speaker checks from time to time that they have been understood. 'Listen before you tell' is a good general rule. There are two types of information giving that have a specific purpose.

1 *Support/feelings* – usually encouraging or congratulatory statements or recognition of feelings. For example, 'Good! That's challenging, but still realistic', or 'I understand you were particularly concerned about . . '. Empathic statements are often helpful in this context: 'I can see that you are concerned about . . '.

2 *Building* – any statement that slightly modifies or adds to any idea or suggestion made. Be accepting, rather than dogmatic – individuals will be more motivated to execute a plan of action if it has been their idea. For example, 'That's a useful suggestion, and you could also use it in next year's objectives'.

Aftermath

It would be exceptional for serious concerns about performance to be first raised in an appraisal. The appraisal itself should be formative. However, both the appraiser and appraisee need to recognise that as registered medical practitioners they must protect patients when they believe that a colleague's health, conduct or performance poses a threat to patients.[3]

Where it becomes apparent, during the appraisal process, that there is a potentially serious performance issue, which requires further discussion or examination, the appraiser must refer the matter immediately to the senior clinician / clinical governance lead and PCT/trust chief executive to take appropriate action. This may, for example, include referral to any support arrangements that may be in place.

The appraiser and appraisee should make arrangements at least once more during the course of the year for around 30 minutes to review progress in relation to the actions and PDP. This could be arranged or resolved via a telephone call rather than an actual meeting.

The senior clinician / clinical governance lead should submit an aggregated and anonymised report on appraisal outcomes, which should be collated and submitted annually to the PCT/trust chief executive. The chief executive should discuss this report with the PCT/trust board. The report must not refer, explicitly or implicitly, to any individuals who have been appraised. The report should highlight emerging training and development needs, organisational or service themes requiring action or investment. It should also review the overall process and operation of the appraisal scheme.

REFERENCES

1 Department of Health. *NHS Appraisal Toolkit.* Available at: www.appraisals.nhs.uk/

2 Chambers R, Wakley G, Field S, *et al. Appraisal for the Apprehensive: a guide for doctors.* Oxford: Radcliffe Publishing; 2003.

3 General Medical Council. *Good Medical Practice.* London: GMC; 2006. paras 26–8.

HOW TO CHAIR A MEETING EFFECTIVELY[1]
What makes a good chair?

Some of these attributes you will have already; others you will need to develop. Think about them as you develop your role and watch other chairs at work. You need the following.

➤ Understanding of the issues and topics being discussed.
➤ Personal knowledge of procedure – for example, standing orders – and of the committee's members.
➤ Strength of character, allowing you to stand your ground and to steer the meeting.
➤ To use your authority – for example, to prevent discussions wandering, stopping those without anything new to add repeating the same point, being able to move on when a point is discussed as far as possible. A chair should be strict without being rude.
➤ Honesty. Being open is the best virtue for a chair. Even though the chair has to stick with the majority decision, the chair will be respected for his/her credibility.
➤ Listening skills.
➤ The ability to sum up the points made in discussions. Before a vote the members must know what they being asked to decide.
➤ Influencing skills and the ability to deal with people outside meetings.

The golden rule of effective chairmanship is to be well prepared. Draft an agenda that reflects the purpose of the meeting. Prioritise items according to importance. Being prepared will enable the chair to guide the meeting in the proper direction rather than allow it to drift aimlessly. Chairmanship is a learned skill; it has to be practised and perfected. It is important to get feedback from others about your ability to chair. Ask others to comment on your strengths and weaknesses.

Running a meeting

Before the meeting starts:
➤ send out the agenda and papers so everyone can read them at least 7 days in advance
➤ book a room and make sure it is easily found
➤ arrange seating to encourage maximum interaction and contribution.

On starting the meeting:
➤ ensure everyone has a copy of the agenda and any papers
➤ ensure you start on time
➤ introduce yourself and welcome all, especially new members
➤ adherance to proper formal meeting procedures by the chair will uphold democratic principles and increase the efficiency and effectiveness of the procedures.

A meeting doesn't just have to involve discussion. Other things that can be done include:
➤ presentations about important developments including slides, overheads, videos and so forth.
➤ outside speakers to talk about issues relevant to the committee
➤ training events
➤ reviews of what has previously been done, congratulating members when

things have been accomplished
➤ bringing refreshments!

On finishing the meeting:
➤ always finish on time
➤ talk with other members about what has been discussed if they wish (much business is conducted outside the formal meeting)
➤ make sure the minutes are written up and circulated to the members within 2 weeks of the meeting.

At the first meeting:
➤ don't talk too much as the chair
➤ don't cover too much
➤ don't have it lasting too long
➤ don't assume everyone has the same knowledge or knows what you are talking about
➤ do get organised in advance
➤ do have a written agenda
➤ do introduce yourselves and make everyone feel comfortable
➤ do think about how to ensure all members can contribute
➤ do have expectations about how members should give input
➤ do enjoy yourself
➤ do finish on time.

At ongoing meetings:
➤ guide by letting members know when discussion has drifted from the topic, usually it will quickly return to it (remind members of the topic and the goals of the meeting)
➤ summarise what less active members have said and link associated points together – accept parts of ideas and ask for them to be developed
➤ spot likely problems – anticipate problems
➤ state the problem in a constructive manner; never blame anyone (agree what decisions the group has to make, do not waste time on other things)
➤ be appropriately humorous – this can convert the most monotonous meeting into a colourful and enjoyable experience
➤ avoid taking sides, becoming too much of a participant in the discussion, manipulating the group towards your own agenda, criticising the values and ideas of others, forcing your own ideas on the group (if necessary have someone else chair the meeting so you can take part), making decisions for the members without asking them for agreement, running late (e.g. by using a timed agenda).

REFERENCE

1 Imperial College Union. *ICU Skills Guide 2005–2006*. London: ICU; 2005. Available at: www.union.ic.ac.uk/resource/skills/chair.html (accessed 24 January 2011).

Index